1,001

NURSING

TIPS & TIMEsavers

Third Edition

Quick and easy tips
for improving patient care

Springhouse Corporation
Springhouse, Pennsylvania

D1092377

STAFF

Executive Director
Matthew Cahill

Editorial Director
June Norris

Art Director
John Hubbard

Managing Editor
David Moreau

Acquisitions Editors
Patricia Kardish Fischer, RN, BSN (project editor); Louise Quinn

Clinical Editor
Collette Bishop Hendler, RN, CCRN

Editors
Margaret Eckman, Ellen Newman

Copy Editors
Cynthia Breuninger (manager), Christine Cunniffe, Mary Durkin, Brenna Mayer

Designers
Arlene Putterman (associate art director), Mary Ludwicki (book designer)

Typographers
Diane Paluba (manager), Joyce Rossi Biletz, Phyllis Marron, Valerie Rosenberger

Production Coordinator
Margaret A. Rastiello

Editorial Assistants
Beverly Lane, Mary Madden, Jeanne Napier

Indexer
Barbara Hodgson

Manufacturing
Deborah Meiris (director), Pat Dorshaw (manager), Anna Brindisi, T.A. Landis

---

Printed in the United States of America.

℞ A member of the Reed Elsevier plc group

TT3E- D N O S A J J M A
02 01 00   10 9 8 7 6 5 4 3

Library of Congress Cataloging-in-Publication Data
 Main entry under title:
 1,001 nursing tips & timesavers
   Rev. ed. of 1,000 nursing tips & timesavers.© 1987.
   "Nursing97 books."
   Includes index.
   1. Nursing—Handbooks, manuals, etc.
 2. Nurses—Time management—Handbooks, manuals, etc. I. Springhouse Corporation. II. 500 nursing tips & timesavers. III. Title: One thousand nursing tips & savers. IV. Title: 1,001 nursing tips and timesavers.
 [DNLM: 1. Nursing—handbooks. WY 18 Z99]
 RT51.A16 1996 610.73   96-69628
 ISBN: 0-87434-850-1

CONTENTS

Foreword

7. Procedures

8. I.V. therapy

9. Medications

10. Safety

11. Cost and timesaver tips

12. Activities of daily living

13. Potpourri

Appendices

Index

FOREWORD

We know how precious a nurse's time is. To help make the most of your valuable time, the editors have collected, reviewed, and organized the best *Tips & Timesavers, Charting Tips,* and *Lab Test Tips* published in the pages of *Nursing* magazine. We've looked for better ways to help you do your work, to save you money, and to make every minute count.

The tips included in this book show how to improve communications and computer skills, perform procedures efficiently, cut costs, administer medications safely, document effectively, and increase your confidence in handling almost any situation.

From the time you spend with patients to the time you spend keeping up with the changing profession, this book will help you save time. That's what *1,001 Nursing Tips & Timesavers* is all about—saving time. And more time is something you can really use, isn't it?

The Editors

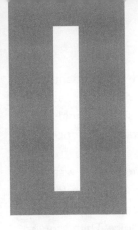

COMMUNICATING

Calling card

I like to make sure my patients know who I am and when I'm available to help them. So, when I'm assigned to patients, I give them an index card on which I've written my name, shift hours, and a brief message encouraging them to call me if they need help or have any questions. I've found this simple device helps me establish a good relationship with all my patients.

LeAnn Chintis, RN

Communicating mats

To make communicating with aphasic patients easier, one nurse illustrated patients' various needs on a placemat. The mat is divided into three sections: activities of daily living, primary needs, and rest and recreation. The activities of daily living section has a toilet, bath, and sink, for example. The rest and recreation section has a radio, bed, and chair.

In all, she illustrated 62 different needs on the 12" x 18" mat. The hospital then had 50 placemats printed and laminated. They're distributed to patients as needed. Using the mat, the patient points to what he wants. Of course, the nursing staff still encourages aphasic patients to communicate on their own. But the mat helps improve communication between the staff and patient, thereby reducing the frustration so common among these patients.

Gail Van Tassell, RN

Sound of the bell

To communicate with a hearing-impaired patient who isn't wearing a hearing aid, place your stethoscope in his ears and speak softly into the bell or diaphragm. This is especially helpful at night because you can talk to the patient without disturbing others on the unit.

Lorraine M. Bearrows, SN

Communicating by computer

When my mother was terminally ill, she couldn't speak because she was on a ventilator. So I bought her a talking alphabet computer toy. The raised letters enabled her to key-stroke her thoughts easily and say good-bye. You can buy this item for under $50 at toy stores.

Caroline E. Nilson, RN, BS

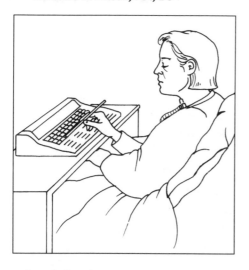

Photo finder

If elderly nursing home patients have trouble finding their rooms, tape a large color photo of the patient's face plus a name card printed in large black letters outside each room. The photo-name cards also help first-time visitors and staff from other departments find specific patients.

Nan Hernikl, RN

Grape juice code

In the hospital where I work, we recently cared for a 14-year-old patient whose many school friends visited constantly. The patient tired easily, but she didn't like to ask her friends to leave so she could rest. To help her, we devised a "grape juice code."

Whenever the patient was tired and wanted her visitors to leave, she'd turn on her call light and ask for some grape juice. Then a nurse would come to her room, tell the visitors that the patient needed to rest, and ask them if they'd mind leaving so she could take a nap. Our code was a success. The patient was spared the embarrassment of asking her friends to leave, yet she got the rest she needed and wanted.

Dixie Burgess, SN

Going for the goal

On our postoperative unit, we have a wipe-off board that's used to record input and output measurements. But I've found another use for it.

I write goals and messages for my patients on the board. For example, I might write, "John will walk in the hall without help three times this shift." I also ask the patient for input on the best goals for that day. At the end of my shift, I draw stars on the board if the patient has accomplished his goals. If he didn't, we decide on the goals for the next day.

This method not only increases a patient's control over his care, but it also helps speed his recovery.

Anna Stuart, RN,C, BSN

Bridging the language gap

Many of our home health care patients don't speak English, and bilingual nurses are in short supply. So we've prepared pages of questions and responses using the most common languages in our area. We leave these pages in the patient's home so the nurse can use them for reference.

She can ask the patient generic questions like, "Where does it hurt?" and "Have you taken your medicine?" Questions specific to the patient's needs are also included.

Bonnie Faherty, RN, CS, PhD

A friendly word

For some of my elderly patients, English is a second language. Their first language is Polish or Italian or German. Although I can't speak these languages, I can communicate with my patients.

On a sheet of paper, I've written some common English words and phrases, with the foreign equivalents opposite them. I post the paper on the patient's bedside bulletin board when he's admitted to my unit. The patients appreciate hearing a friendly "good morning" in their own language: gin dobre (Polish),

buon giorno (Italian), guten morgen (German). They also respond appreciatively when they're told it's time to eat, take medicine, or turn to the side.

Fe Perez, RN

In the cards

When I have trouble communicating with a patient who doesn't speak English, I use a set of picture cards that I've made. These cards show foods (to help with menu selection), medications, and objects related to personal care (toothbrush, shower, toilet). Communicating this way reduces frustration for both of us.

Robbin McNamara, RN, BSN

Ready reference for tetanus injection

When I give a tetanus injection to a patient, I suggest that he put a small piece of tape with the day's date on the back of his health insurance card. That way, he'll have a handy reminder of when he received the injection.

Kim Leighton, RN

Admission timesaver

To help patients who can't read, we've recorded information they need to know about admission—in English and Spanish—on cassette tapes. This includes the admission consent form and preoperative

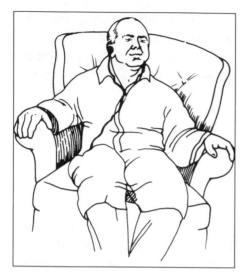

teaching booklet. After the patient listens to the tape, a nurse answers his questions and assesses how well he understood the information. This process saves time for us and embarrassment for the patient. Also, he can replay parts of the tape if necessary.

Susan McCormic, RN

ECGs to go

When a patient is discharged from our coronary care unit, we give him a copy of his last electrocardiogram (ECG) rhythm strip and suggest he carry it in his wallet. It could save him an unnecessary hospital admission later.

For instance, at some future time the patient may have another ECG run that shows some abnormalities he's being treated for. If his regular doctor isn't available to interpret the results, another doctor might want to admit him to determine whether these abnormalities are new or old findings. The rhythm strip in his wallet will provide the information immediately, and the patient won't have to be admitted.

May Edwards, RN

Questions for callers

At the urgent-care center where I work, we receive many phone inquiries. So I made a list of questions for the receptionist to ask when patients call with symptoms.

For example, if the call is about chest pain, she'll ask for the duration of pain, intensity, and location. This way, she can report pertinent information to me or the doctor.

Robbin McNamara, RN, BSN

Special delivery

As a prenatal class instructor, I enjoy getting to know my students in the 6 weeks we spend together. And I try not to lose touch when the course ends. I keep a list of my students' names and phone numbers, and I check the local newspaper daily for birth announcements. A few days after each baby is born, I call the new parents to congratulate them. They appreciate the follow-up call and enjoy sharing their labor and delivery experiences.

Wendy Kaveney, RN, BSN

Patient information

Note of confidence
Sometimes a patient scheduled for arthroscopic surgery may be afraid that the wrong knee or shoulder will be operated on. So before surgery, I cut a 6" to 7" strip of silk tape and write on it with a bright marker: "NOT THIS LEG—THE OTHER ONE," for example. Then I put the message across the healthy leg. This visual aid makes the patient feel more confident, and it reduces his anxiety.
Dorothy Fisk, RN

Power of pictures
To reduce the number of Medicare denials for home nursing care, we use photographs to document a patient's need for wound care.

First, we obtain written permission from patients to photograph wounds that will need extensive— and costly—treatment. Then, we take two photos of the affected area, keeping a copy of one in the patient's chart. The originals are sent to Medicare with the patient's claim form. If necessary, we photograph the wound later to document healing.
Sr. Roberta Downey, RN

Helpful stick figures
To remind myself of patients' special restrictions and needs, I include stick figure drawings in their charts.

On the drawings, I indicate any invasive devices (such as an I.V. line or nasogastric tube) and surgical openings (such as a stoma or tracheostomy) my patients have.

Just a quick look at the drawings makes it easier to remember how restricted some patients can be and how much they need a little extra attention.
Mimi Prenger, RN

Procedure cards: Simple reminders
We have float, per diem, and agency nurses working on our medical-surgical unit. To maintain consistency and quality assurance, we've developed reminder cards for administering total parenteral nutrition or peripheral parenteral nutrition. These cards, which include key points of the procedures, are left at the patient's bedside.
Donna Duff, RN

Body language
When we chart information on a patient with a pressure sore, we use a black ink stamp showing the outline of the human body. Then we circle the location of the pressure sore; label it for size, stage, and drainage; and describe other significant characteristics (such as redness, edema, and odor). We use

the stamp on nurses' notes, care plans, treatment Kardex, admission forms, transfer forms, and discharge plans. This charting aid quickly communicates important information.

Ann Dodge, RN, ET

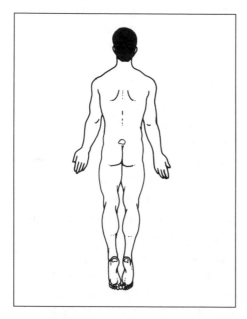

Last bottle

If a patient being discharged from our recovery room is on his last I.V. bottle, we indicate it by taping a bandage and an alcohol wipe to the bottle. This lets the patient's nurse know that the I.V. line can be removed after the bottle is finished.

Maryann Ganci, RN
Sue Greba, LPN

Bedside reminder

During report, we keep 2" square pieces of tape on our clipboards, and we list on them the things we'll need to do for our patients. After report, we put the tape on each patient's bedside table, where it serves as a handy reminder, saving a lot of trips to the Kardex.

Marsha Mohr, RN, BSN
Linette Seamon, RN, BSN

Specimen collection reminder

On our coronary care unit, we sometimes inadvertently disposed of urine or stool when a specimen was needed. We solved this problem by hanging a single cork tile on the door to the rest room. We tack urinalysis and stool specimen laboratory slips and Hemoccult reminders to the cork. That way, we all remember to collect the specimens.

Joyce W. McBride, RN, CCRN

Ready reference for medication requests

In our busy rehabilitation unit, I'm often in one place while the nursing assistants are in another. When a patient requests a medication, a nursing assistant will use a spiral notebook on my desk to write down the patient's room number and name and the time. I check the notebook every 5 minutes, then enter the time I give the patient any medication. (Of course, I also enter this information on the patient's medication Kardex.)

This not only serves as a means of communication between the nursing assistants and me, but also saves time for all of us. And it works as a reference to find out when a patient received medication.

Isabelle Ann Kazmierczak, LPN

Dropping a note

To save time in my geriatric unit, I carry a small pad of sticky-backed notepaper. If I need to communicate routine patient information to a nursing assistant and she's not available, I just leave a note on the patient's door, along with the date and time. For example, I might write, "Please force fluids for Mr. Green." This system works well and my staff always reports back to me regarding the notes.

Connie M. Harris, LPN

Computing signs

In our unit, we post a sign on a patient's door or in his room to notify staff members of procedures in progress, tests that need to be done, and so on. Each time we need a sign, I print it on my computer and copy it for our files. By doing the signs on the computer, I can quickly revise them or add specific instructions (such as the time the patient's weight should be taken).

Bonnie Hermesman, RN,C, BSN

Prominent profiles

On our busy medical unit, we've come up with a way to prominently display patient profiles. We write essential information about each patient in bold letters on five strips of heavy paper or posterboard. (Or you can cut up a manila folder.) Then we insert the strips into the sleeves on a partitioned sheet of plastic. The sheet is then tacked above the patient's bed.

The information we write on the strips includes: (1) the patient's name, doctor, and teaching team (symbolized by different colored dots); (2) dietary information; (3) fluid restrictions; (4) general care instructions and precautions; and (5) physical limitations. If orders change or a patient is discharged, the strips are removed and filed.

Bonnie L. Guith, RN, MS

FORMulating shift report

When I was a new staff nurse on a medical-surgical unit, I was surprised and frustrated with all the note-taking expected of me during shift report. Having to write name, room number, diagnosis, vital signs, and so on for patient after patient took a lot of time and kept me from listening attentively to report. So, with suggestions from my coworkers, I designed a form for use during report that looks something like the one shown at the top of the next page:

Room		
Patient		
Dx		
IV/I&O		
VS		
Treaments		
Lab results		

The form was enthusiastically adopted by nurses on my unit. It can easily be altered to reflect specific needs on any nursing unit.

Sandra D. Andrew, RN, BS

Color coding for DNR orders

At the skilled nursing facility where I work, we use yellow or pink to indicate a patient's code status.

If the patient has a do-not-resuscitate (DNR) order, we use a yellow marker to color the name label on the back of his chart. We also color his ID band yellow. But if the patient wants to be resuscitated, we color the name label and band pink.

Of course, the ID band is just one additional way of alerting us to a patient's code status.

Alice T. Morell, RN

Tab for DNR order

Here's what we do on our unit for fast access to a patient's do-not-resuscitate (DNR) order.

When the doctor writes a DNR order, we make a tab from a piece of tape and place it on the right side of the order; the tab extends about ½" from the page. Anyone can easily locate the order, including the attending doctor, nurses, and the unit secretary. And the tape can be pulled off if the code status changes or the patient is transferred.

Kimberly Barker, RN, BSN

Easy access to patient information

Try this system for organizing printouts of computerized patient care plans.

Staple all of the printouts together in the upper left-hand corner. Fold down the upper right-hand corner of the first page of each patient's care plan. Then write the patient's name and room number on this corner. Now you'll be able to find the information you want without sifting through a stack of papers.

Mary Kautzer, Unit Secretary

Color-coded information

A tricolor pen really helps me keep my patient information organized. During change-of-shift report, I write the previous shift report in red ink on the patient profile sheets. After assessing each patient, I write my information in black ink. If any changes occur during my shift, I note them on the profile in green ink. This makes charting, updating a doctor on a patient's condition, and giving end-of-shift report easier and more comprehensive.

Elizabeth M. Champlin, RN, BSN

Report sheets: Passing the baton

Whenever a nurse leaves our unit for lunch or a break, she gives the report sheets for her patients to a colleague. This way, if a patient's relative or attending doctor has questions, another nurse can answer them.

Leah McNulty, RN, BSN

Patient transfer: In the cards

A patient may be transferred several times during his hospitalization. But the nurse who's assigned to transfer the patient may have never cared for him. So she might not be familiar with his history.

To make sure the nurse doesn't overlook important information during the transfer report, we've started filling out a history card for each of our patients. This is a simple index card that contains the patient's history, chief admitting complaint, major tests, and changes in his condition. It's placed in the patient's Kardex, and it can easily be updated as his condition changes.

We've found that since we've been using the history card, transfers are smoother and report time is shorter.

Mary E. Fassetta, RN, MS

Out with the list...in with the form

To save time in the morning during shift changes, we created a form that lists our unit's room and bed numbers. Each morning, one of the nurses circles the room and bed numbers of patients who need to be weighed and indicates those who need finger-stick blood glucose monitoring. Then she posts the form for everyone to see. This way, nurses don't have to make a list of what each patient needs every day.

Julie R. Welsh, RN, MS

Discharge at a glance

At the hospital where I work, four or more doctors may be consulting on a patient's care. So when a patient is discharged, we take the name label from the front of his chart and place it on the counter at the nurses' station. When the doctors make their rounds, they can tell at a glance which patients have been discharged. This saves time for them and also for us.

Carol Harrison, RN

With significant others

"Baby-grams" for parents

If babies in the neonatal intensive care unit are brought in from rural areas, their parents have to travel long distances to visit or make expensive phone calls.

Keep parents posted on their baby's progress by sending "baby-grams" on inexpensive postcards. On the card's message side, put the baby's footprint and a short note "from the baby."

The note can state the baby's weight and say something positive about his condition, if only to describe his curly hair or lusty cry. Parents love getting these cards and can add them to their baby books.

Nancy Hogg, RN

Dear Mom and Dad, 🙂

Today I gained 2 ounces. I am also learning to cry loud enough when I am hungry so my nurses hear me. Miss you.

Love,
Thomas

Familiar faces

We hang photographs of each staff member in our critical care unit right outside the unit's doors, under the heading "These are the people who will be caring for you." We also list each person's name and position under her photo. This "minigallery" helps patients and visitors feel more comfortable when entering the unit.

Elizabeth Ray, RN, CCRN, MSN

Calming calls

Family visits should have a calming influence on seriously ill patients, but in many cases they have the opposite effect. One obvious reason: an anxious family transmits its anxiety to the patient.

Ask doctors what they want the families of their patients to know. Then relay that information to the family on their next visit. Or, adopt the same routine, except phone each family every morning, telling them how the patient spent the night and what the doctor had to say.

Catherine Baden, RN, BS

Caring after death

Nurses at Hospice Nana in Bristol, N.H., don't stop caring after one of their patients dies. Instead, they make bereavement visits to the family 1, 2, and 3 weeks after the patient's death, then at 3 months, 6 months, and 1 year. They also visit at other times if they think the family needs it.

The hospice nurses have found that many families experience health-related problems within 6 months after a patient's death. That's when the cards have stopped coming, visits from friends have become less frequent, and the death is supposed to be "a thing of the past." But family members whose time was consumed by caring for the terminally ill person find the loneliness difficult to bear. They become depressed and predisposed to illness.

The visits have helped the nurses offset this loneliness and have enabled the nurses to detect illnesses early. For instance, nurses have detected hypertension that developed in a widow 6 months after her husband died and severe depression in a mother whose child died of leukemia.

The nurses welcome the chance to support the family throughout the year following the patient's death—and families welcome the support and preventive health care they receive.

M. Dolan, RN

Staff information

Sign of efficiency
On our postanesthesia care unit, we placed a brightly colored "NEXT" sign over the cubicle that is empty. This way, the circulating nurse, doctor, or anesthetist entering our unit knows right away where to take the next patient.

Lucinda S. Powers, RN, BSN

Across the board
To keep everyone on our unit aware of patient assignments, we've set up an erasable board listing each patient's name, room number, and the nurse assigned to him for each shift. At a glance, nurses and other health care professionals working on the unit can identify the nurse assigned to a particular patient.

Charge nurses have found the board helpful when making change-of-shift reports or planning new assignments.

Linda Tate, RN, BSN

Stick to it
As a clinical instructor, I've found a good way to keep track of Kardex cards and charts when my students are using them: I ask the students to replace each card or chart they borrow with a sticky-backed note. The note includes the student's name and where she's taking the card or chart.

This method works on medication cards, too. A note alerts staff nurses that students are giving those medications that day.

Judy Cummings, RN, MS

A show of lights
When our hospital was remodeled, a light system was installed on each unit to make locating staff members easier. Whenever we enter a room, we press a color-coded button. A corresponding colored light goes on outside the room, above the door. On our unit, we use one color for staff nurses and another for the charge nurse. The lights are all visible from the nurses' station.

Catherine Piccinni, RN

Color-coded cart

The last time I used our pediatric crash cart, I found that much of the needed equipment was either missing or the wrong size. So after the code, I started to organize the cart. I came across a Broselow Tape, which is divided into sections. Each section is a different color and contains information on pediatric drug dosages and equipment sizes. You run the tape from the top of the child's head to the bottom of his feet. Then you look at the color

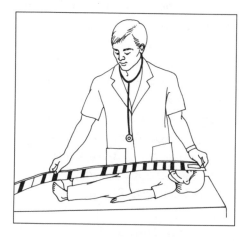

where the feet are and you use the drug and equipment information printed in that color block to treat the child.

After studying the tape, I decided to paint the drawers of the pediatric code cart to match its colors. Then I stocked each drawer with the appropriate equipment. I also color-coded bags of respiratory supplies and placed them in the respiratory supply box on top of the crash cart.

Now after measuring a child with the Broselow Tape, we can immediately open the correct drawer—and have the equipment we need at our fingertips.

Darlene Portelance, RN, CEN

Listen for the beep

We use a beeper system to locate a nurse anywhere on our unit. Here's how it works: Each nurse carries a beeper that's tied into the unit's call light system. When a patient's call light goes on, the unit secretary answers, then transmits a signal to alert the patient's nurse. The nurse who is being paged can identify the patient's room number by pressing a button. If she's busy with another patient, she can signal the unit secretary to send someone else to check on the patient.

This system also allows us to transmit numerical messages to our nurses. For example, "0000" means "Come to the nurses' station."

Liz Lawrence, RN

Moving target

Here's how I make myself easily accessible to the unit secretary during my night shift in a 20-bed antepartum unit: I keep my supplies on a small cart and leave it outside each patient's room while on my rounds. This way, she can quickly look down the hall and locate me instantly.

Lisa Wilson, RN

Saving time with a bell

I used to work on a unit that had three long hallways leading away from the nurses' station. Searching for the nurse who had the keys to the narcotics cabinet took a lot of time, so we came up with a solution. We placed a bell on the counter at the nurses' station. If someone needed the keys, she'd just ring the bell and the nurse who had them would come to the nurses' station.

If she couldn't leave her patient, she'd use the intercom in the patient's room to tell the nurse who needed the keys where she was.

Tammy Ferrin, RN, BSN

Expert advice

You may be using a variety of medical devices and equipment with which you're unfamiliar. Make a list of those items, then next to each, note one or more staff members who are experts at using the equipment. Post the list on each unit. When someone runs into trouble, she'll know whom to call.

Edwina A. McConnell, RN, Phd

Float notes

To help float nurses on our unit, we've printed notes describing our nursing routines and procedures. The notes save time by answering commonly asked questions. They help the float nurses feel less anxious, and they also promote consis-

tent nursing care.

Jeanne M. Albertini, RN

Needed numbers

We tape the materials-management order numbers for defibrillator pads, electrocardiogram machine paper, and electrodes to the defibrillator. This makes it easy for the person who uses these supplies in an emergency or who finds them missing during daily code cart checks to replace them. All she has to do is look at the defibrillator for the order numbers, not hunt through the supply book.

Julie R. Welsh, RN, MS

Prepared for an emergency

At the small hospital where I work, we call a "code 238"—the telephone extension for the obstetric unit—when we need more staff to help out with an emergency cesarean. And to make sure we have the right supplies to prepare the woman for surgery, we stock a code 238 tray with items we'll need, such as indwelling urinary catheters and I.V. equipment.

Louise Coull, RN

Pocket full of charts

Whenever I find useful charts, such as advanced cardiac life support algorithms, I reduce them on a photocopying machine. I mount the charts on index cards, laminate the cards, and secure them with a ring through the top. Now I have an inexpensive pocket resource that's small enough to carry with me during my shift.

Katie Morales, RN

Messages from the heart

On the progressive care unit where I work, we fill a heart-shaped basket with blank, heart-shaped pieces of paper. When we want to send a message (like "thanks," "cheer up," or "good job") to a coworker or patient, we write it on one of these papers. This boosts morale and can brighten someone's day.

Valerie Messina, RN, MSN

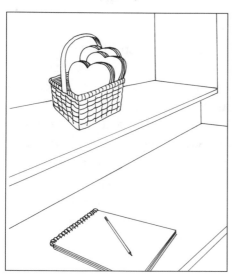

Morale booster

On our unit, we don't let compliments slip by. We write them down in our "Positive Comments" notebook. Staff members pen thank-you's for help received; patients and family members note their apprecia-

tion of our efforts. We keep the notebook in a central location so we can read it, p.r.n. It's a real morale booster.

Pam Bartley, RN

A good book

When I'm feeling depressed, I take out a notebook I call "My Strokes." I've included notes, memos, and letters written by my coworkers and managers to congratulate me on jobs well done. I've also compiled my own list of accomplishments. These reminders of good work never fail to put me in a better mood when I'm feeling down.

Audrey Gilmore, RN, C

Color-coded convenience

In our busy medical-surgical unit, we have a color-coded board in the nurses' station highlighting our services and identifying physicians by specialty. Each specialty has its own color—for example, cardiothoracic is red, urology is blue, and orthopedics is green. Each physician's name and pager number is highlighted on the board in the color corresponding to his specialty. This way, when a nurse needs to page a physician in an emergency, she can quickly find his number.

Carol A. Housler, RN

Nursing network

To meet nurses from other units in the hospital, try hosting a networking function on your unit. Set aside a day every few months for one of these get-togethers. (An ice cream party is great for summer months.) Make sure nurses on each shift are included. These networking parties will give you a chance to share knowledge and support each other—important steps toward quality patient care and job satisfaction.

Amy Jennewine Van Gulick, RN, OCN, BSN

Glads for grads

During spring orientation, I give each new graduate nurse a few gladiolus bulbs to plant at home. I tell the graduates that when the bulbs have grown into flowers, each of them will have grown comfortable in her new nursing role.

Beth Weaver, RN,C, BSN

Good reading

Our hospital has a great way to notify staff nurses of important events, such as staff-development workshops, unit meetings, or continuing education classes. Notices are posted on bulletin boards located on the inside doors of staff rest rooms.

Deborah L. Anderson, RN

2 TEACHING

Printed pointers for parents

At the hospital where I work, a new mother receives a lot of information (such as breast-feeding and car safety films, bath demonstrations, nutrition lectures) in a short time—especially if she's discharged within 24 hours after delivery. It's no wonder, then, that she's overwhelmed with all these new facts, figures, and explanations to remember.

We made up a folder to send home with the mother that contains information on parenting: resources such as the LaLeche League, for instance; a sheet with practical information such as cord care, how to take the baby's temperature, and what to do if the baby is fussy, has diarrhea, or is vomiting; and a sheet describing the mother's physical condition during the postpartum period. New mothers appreciate the folder because it reinforces what we've already discussed with them during their short stay in the hospital.

Teresa Hays, RN

A balloon bust

We needed a breast model for our prenatal breast-feeding classes that was portable, pliable, realistic, *and* inexpensive. A small, inflated, oblong balloon met all these criteria.

The end of the balloon represents a nipple. (Or if we want to show a flat nipple, we hold the inflated balloon in the middle and force the air to the end.) We can demonstrate nipple preparation exercises and how to use a breast pump on our balloon breast model. And we always get a laugh when we pull out a green, orange, or multicolored breast model.

Janet E. Marshman, RN

Demo doll

To teach patients and new staff nurses how to care for a Hickman catheter, we use the chest cover from an old resuscitation manikin. We can simulate all Hickman catheter care procedures on the manikin: exit-site care, flushing, blood drawing, changing the injection cap, and clamping. Both staff and patients appreciate this "live" demonstration of Hickman catheter care much more than the textbook presentation we previously gave.

Pat Tobin, RN

Labeling drug samples

In the doctor's office where I work, we frequently give patients sample drugs until they can get their prescriptions filled. The samples, although clearly marked with the drug's name, don't have orders for how or when the drugs should be taken.

To help these patients remember how to take their new drugs, I devised this system: I place the sample in a small paper bag and attach a 2" x 4" label on the outside of the bag. On the label I write the date, the patient's name, the drug's name, its strength, when to take the drug, and what it's for. The label reinforces the verbal instructions the patient gets in the office.

As an added help, I staple a card with the patient's next appointment date to the folded bag. Now all his medical information is together in one place.

Lori Gross, RN

Group therapy

On our busy general surgical floor, we usually are only able to give brief *individual* preoperative instructions to our patients. But we supplement these individual conferences with a group session.

On the evening before their surgery, we invite patients to the lounge and ask them to bring their pillows and inhalation spirometers. After discussing basic preoperative events, we have the patients practice coughing and deep breathing. We also demonstrate the proper use of spirometers and how to splint incisions with pillows.

Besides ensuring that our patients know what to expect the next day, the group sessions also give them the chance to share their feelings about surgery and to encourage each other.

Donna Avallone, RN

Well-read

In the rehabilitation unit where I work, patient teaching starts with reading. I give each patient a book or article about his illness to help him understand his condition and participate in his care.

Fe Perez, RN

Bridging the gap with pictures

At the hospital where I work, we recently had to teach home care to a Spanish-speaking mother. Although she was ready to be discharged, her baby still needed some medication. None of the weekend staff nurses spoke Spanish, but we didn't want to wait until Monday to start our teaching. So we decided to communicate nonverbally—we used pictures to indicate when each medication was to be given.

First, we drew clock faces across a piece of paper. Then we drew the clock hands to indicate the time for each feeding and medication dose. (The baby had to be fed every 3 hours, and she needed medication every 6 hours.) We indicated the difference between a.m. and p.m. by drawing a sun or a moon above the clock.

We cut small pieces of colored tape to correspond to each medication (for example, green for ergocalciferol); white tape was used to indicate formula. Then we labeled each medicine bottle and syringe with the corresponding colored tape. We placed the correct tape colors under the clock for the times the medications and formula were to be given.

On Monday, a Spanish-speaking nurse reported that the baby's mother understood our teaching. She was more relaxed about feeding and administering medication—and we were more confident that the baby would receive proper care at home.

Sarah Oldham, RN

Pictorial approach to charting intake

I've devised a pictorial chart that pediatric patients and patients who don't speak English can use to keep an accurate record of soft food and liquid intake.

The chart is divided into columns, with clock faces visually illustrating each hour of a nursing shift. Pictures of liquid or soft food items—milk, ice cream, juice, soda, gelatin, and water—are included in each column. The patient simply checks off or colors in whatever he ate or drank during the time period.

Selina Hays, SN

Note board: Getting the message

You can use a dry erase message board in a patient's room to write notes to him and reminders about patient-teaching tips. (The board is especially helpful when caring for a patient with dementia or Alzheimer's disease.)

Diane Warwick, SN, CNA

Video reminder: In the cards

I've developed reminder cards that encourage patients to view patient-education videos on our hospital's closed-circuit television station.

On a 3" x 5" index card, I write the topic (for example, smoking, nutrition, heart disease) and the days and times the video for that topic will be shown. When a patient is admitted, his nurse pulls the appropriate card from a file box and places it on his care plan. She gives him the card on the day the video is scheduled to be shown. After he views the video, he gives the card back to her and she documents what he's seen.

Sharon Britt, RN,C

Bigger type

At our home care agency, we instruct diabetic patients on meal planning. When we copy printed literature on the subject to give to our patients, we adjust the copier to increase the print size. Because many diabetics have poor eyesight, this helps them read the information that's so important to our teaching.

Joyce E. Heil, RN, BSN

Keeping patients TRIM

At our hospital, we've adopted the TRIM teaching method to make sure our patients can care for themselves at home. For example, here's what we tell a patient with congestive heart failure:

• **T**reatment—Check weight weekly.
• **R**estrictions—Eliminate salt and salted foods. Avoid extremes of heat, humidity, and cold. Don't exercise strenuously, but walk 1 mile a day. Schedule daily rest periods.
• **I**mpending signs and symptoms—Report swelling of hands or feet, shortness of breath, or weight gain of 3 pounds or more per week to your doctor.

• **M**edications—digoxin, 0.25 mg, four times a day; furosemide, 40 mg, twice a day; potassium chloride, 30 mEq, four times a day. Take all medications as directed. Report any adverse reactions to your doctor.

Sandra Dearholt, RN, CCRN, BSN
Teresa Gentry, RN, BSN

Understanding a "no seeds" diet

A simple analogy explains why a patient with diverticulosis can't eat seeds. I compare a seed getting caught in the intestines with a seed getting caught under dentures. The patient can understand the pain, inflammation, and possible infection that might cause. And I tell him that although he could remove the dentures and seed, treatment for a seed lodged in the intestines isn't as easy.

This analogy isn't completely accurate medically, but it's quickly grasped and it reinforces the "no seeds" diet.

Elissa Sommer, RN

Fruitless practice

With today's high cost of food, using grapefruit and oranges for practicing intramuscular and subcutaneous injections isn't practical.

But we've found a suitable substitute: a package of the blue gel that can be frozen and used to cool food in picnic hampers.

We can puncture the unfrozen package repeatedly, and it doesn't leak. We can also pinch it up or spread it for realistic injection practicing. The packages come in various sizes, but we've found the smallest size most useful.

Jeanne Sorrell, RN, MS

Wet wafer: Blow it dry

The skin under a patient's ileostomy or colostomy wafer may itch if the wafer gets wet. And if the patient scratches, the pouch could come loose. So tell him to blow cool air from a hair dryer on the wafer. This will dry the area and help to prevent problems.

Joan Jacoby, SN

Covering casts

I suggest that patients with a fiberglass leg or arm cast cover the cast with a nylon knee sock to prevent it from tearing clothing, furniture, and bedding. If the patient has a leg cast, the sock will keep his toes warm and clean. If he has an arm cast, tell

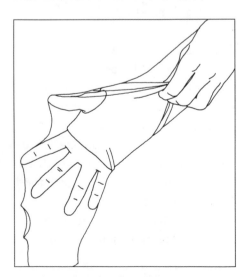

him to cut the sock at the end so his fingers won't be covered.

These socks are inexpensive, and they can be washed or replaced as needed.

Betsy Beinlich, RN

Teaching self-catheterization to the elderly

Our visiting nurse agency has many patients over age 65. Teaching them self-catheterization can be a challenge. Here's what we do.

We tell the patient to attach the red rubber end of the catheter directly to a leg bag before inserting the catheter into his urethra. After catheter insertion, the urine flows into the leg bag, so the patient doesn't have to worry about aiming the catheter end into a receptacle. This method is especially helpful if the patient has poor mobility or coordination or if he can only use one hand adequately. If he has poor eyesight or hearing, you can tell him to feel the catheter to sense the warmth as the urine begins to flow.

Jane Marie Brown, RN

Practice paste

Patients can practice measuring the correct dose of nitroglycerin ointment by using toothpaste instead of nitroglycerin. This is easy and less expensive than using the actual medication. Plus, you won't have to worry about the patient possibly harming himself by getting the ointment on his fingers.

Cathleen M. Burrage, RN, BSN

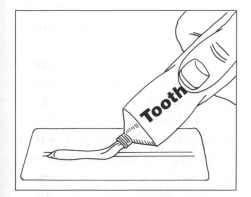

Don't forget to document

When you teach your patient about his medication during administration times, make sure to document this as formal patient teaching. Initially assess his familiarity with the medication and give him a basic explanation of the drug's action. You can even give him an information card about his medications for his wallet, including indications, mechanisms of action, dosage information, adverse effects, and drug interactions. During subsequent administrations, further assess and reinforce his understanding of the drug, remembering to document this as well.

Karen Teves Frazier, RN

Warnings to remember

When teaching my patients the warning signs of a possible stroke, I find this mnemonic helpful: **We kNow** the **H**ints to a **P**ossible **S**troke. **We** can **S**ee the **D**ifference. The phrase helps my patients remember to be on the lookout for:

Weakness
Numbness
Headache
Personality changes
Speech changes
Sight changes
Dizziness.

Tammy Mertes, SN

Infection detection

Discharge instructions may be overwhelming to patients who are leaving the emergency department after being treated for abrasions or lacerations. To make sure they remember the signs of infection, just remind them that "**P**eople **S**hould **R**eally **H**elp **P**eople":

Pain
Swelling
Redness
Heat
Pus.

This easy-to-remember mnemonic will help them learn what signs to report to the doctor.

Eileen M. Suraci, RN

Daily dose: Circled reminder

I always write down a sample medication schedule on a patient's discharge summary form. Then I circle the times the patient has already received medication that day. Once he gets home, he'll know when he needs to take his next dose.

Theresa M. Dando, RN, BSN

A drug tip-off

To help ensure that patients comply with their medication regimens at home, I keep a file of "drug tips." For example: Bactrim should be taken with a full glass of water, and the patient should drink plenty of water during the day.

When a patient is being discharged, I review with him the tips for his medications. If the patient is elderly or forgetful, I review the tips with a family member, too. Then, I write the tips on a card for the patient to take home with him. Even if these tips are printed on the drug containers, my teaching serves as one more way to ensure compliance.

Marianne Anderson, LPN

A proposition

Next time you give a patient a sheet of discharge instructions for a self-treatment procedure (such as stoma care, insulin injection, or colostomy irrigation), make sure the instructions are written step-by-step in large, block letters and are clearly numbered. Paste the instructions to the front of an 8" x 10" cardboard, easel-type picture frame. The patient can set the instructions in front of him and won't have to strain to

read small print.

Marie O'Toole, RN, MSN

Handy logbook

We log telephone calls from discharged patients in a notebook we keep at the nurses' station. Included are the patient's name, diagnosis, topic discussed, advice given, and length of the call. This information helps us spot weaknesses in discharge teaching and maintain a record of time spent on calls. We could also use the book as evidence if a patient ever sued one of us for malpractice.

Marcy Meitzner, RN

Homework for patients

Patient teaching can be a challenge if you're giving a lot of information in a limited amount of time. Here's what I do to enhance my teaching:

Before I give a patient his education pamphlet, I underline the important information in red ink. Then I tell him that his homework is to read the material so we can discuss it the next day. If I'm demonstrating a procedure to the patient, I ask him to practice before I meet with him again.

Presenting the material as a homework assignment stresses the importance of learning. It also makes the patient more responsible for his own care.

Julie R. Welsh, RN, MS

Travel plans

A patient who must leave your unit for X-rays or tests might be anxious about what's in store for him. Before you send him on his way, tell him a little bit about the department he'll be visiting and the scheduled tests. And to make sure he'll feel comfortable, encourage him to use the bathroom before he leaves your unit and to wear socks or slippers. You might want to give him a blanket in case he has to wait a while in a drafty hallway. Above all, assure him that the health care workers he'll meet will take good care of him and will be glad to answer any questions.

Mary H. Cho, RN

Senior class tips

In a course on aging, I learned some tips that might be helpful to other nurses working with geriatric patients.

For example, patients who have poor eyesight may have trouble reading your patient education handouts if you use blue paper. Use nonglare, yellow paper instead. Or if yellow paper isn't available, use a yellow highlighter to emphasize important points. If possible, have your printed materials enlarged so the letters, numbers, and words are easier to read.

Finally, because some of your patients may have a problem with short-term memory, frequently review and reinforce the points in your lesson.

Kay Preshlock, RN, BS

Cardiac rehab: In the cards

At the hospital where I work, we follow a seven-step cardiac rehabilitation program. To promote continuity of care and to give us a quick reference tool, we've typed up and laminated cards that describe the patient activity and education for each step. The appropriate card is placed in the patient's Kardex each day.

Deb Falk, RN

REDUCE risks with a mnemonic

I've devised this simple mnemonic to teach patients how to reduce their risk of atherosclerosis:

- **R**ed meat should be limited to 3 to 4 ounces a day.
- **E**xercise or engage in some activity.
- **D**o listen to your doctor.
- **U**se less salt while cooking or at the table.
- **C**holesterol should be below 200 mg/dl.
- **E**at less fried food and more vegetables.

Stacy C. Hoffman, SN

Customized medication cards

Create customized medication cards for your patients who take several medications so that you can easily keep track of prescriptions and dosages. Just type your patient's medication information in neat columns, reduce the list to business-card size by using a copy machine, and then laminate the card with self-laminating sheets.

Encourage your patient to keep the card in his wallet.

Mary Jo Early

Drug	Dosage	Indication
Zestril	20mg– 1 tab–a.m.	blood pressure
Norvasc	5 mg– ½ tab–p.m.	blood pressure
aspirin	81 mg– 1 tab–a.m.	blood thinner
Minitran patch	0.2 mg/hr on a.m.– off p.m.	heart
Nitrostat	$\frac{1}{150}$ gr– 1 tab under tongue, p.r.n.	chest pain

The diabetic patient

Diabetes analogy: Street talk

For some patients, we use analogies to explain the pathophysiology of diabetes. We tell them to think of the body's blood vessels as streets, the cells as garages, the sugar as cars, and insulin as the driveways that allow cars to get from the streets into the garages.

In type I, insulin-dependent diabetes, the pancreas doesn't produce the insulin needed to carry sugar from the blood into the cells. The analogy for the patient: The cars (sugar) stay on the street (blood vessels) because there aren't any driveways (insulin).

In type II, non-insulin-dependent diabetes, where insulin is produced but meets resistance at the cellular level, we use this analogy: The driveways (insulin) are there, but the garage doors (cells) are closed. Because there's too much fat inside the cells, only so many cars (sugar) will fit into the garages (cells). The rest stay on the streets (blood vessels).

Corinne C. Harmon, RN, MS
John Hamby, PhD

Hand it to them

When one of my diabetic patients must do daily fingersticks for blood glucose monitoring, I give him the outline of a pair of hands traced on a piece of paper. The patient can mark the site where he took his last blood sample. This helps him to remember to rotate sites, preventing sore fingers.

Claudia Boss, SN

Practice shots

To help diabetic patients become more confident about giving themselves insulin injections, try this: Fold an elastic bandage to a thickness greater than the length of an insulin syringe needle. Tape it to the patient's skin at the site where he'll give the real injection later. Let him practice "sticking" the elastic bandage, using a sterile insulin syringe and a vial of sterile water.

Kirsten Rutherford-Harris, RN

Let your V be your guide

Recently, I was teaching a blind diabetic patient how to administer her insulin. When practicing, she'd often miss the injection site and stick her fingers (which were holding the skin taut) instead.

So I made an injection guide by taping two tongue blades together at one end to form a V. Then, just before she was ready to inject herself, she placed the tongue blades on her thigh, felt the outline of the blades, and inserted the needle—right on target—inside the V.

Theresa Gilliland, RN

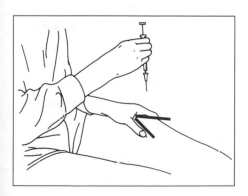

Practice pad

Teaching a newly diagnosed diabetic patient to fill a syringe is usually easy. But teaching him to inject the insulin is another story—jabbing the needle into the skin is scary. So, to help patients learn this technique, use an injection practice pad.

Place a foam rubber sponge, measuring 6" x 8" x 1 ½", between two sheets of clear plastic about 1" larger than the sponge. Seal the edges of the plastic with tape. Then punch holes in the reinforced edges on each end and insert strings for ties. Finally, cut a large target hole in the plastic on one side. Then tie the pad snugly around the patient's upper thigh.

Using 0.5 ml of sterile water instead of insulin, the patient can practice injecting the needle through the sponge until he learns the proper direction and force. Placing the pad on his thigh also lets him practice at an actual injection site.

Make these pads in adults' and children's sizes and include one in each teaching kit supplied for diabetics by the central service department.

Marjorie B. Shaljean, RN

Rotation reminder

When teaching a newly diagnosed diabetic patient the importance of rotating injection sites, reinforce your lesson by marking the sites with a povidone-iodine swab. Because the povidone-iodine eventually washes off, give your patient a site rotation card as a *constant* reminder of his last injection site.

Elisa B. Bachrow, LPN

Food for thought

When I teach diabetic patients about diet, one thing we discuss is the importance of measuring food portions. I suggest that they make model portions out of modeling clay to represent serving sizes of ¼, ⅓, ½, ⅔, ¾, and 1 cup. They can put these on a cookie sheet. Then, when they prepare meals, they can compare each serving to the appropriate model to estimate the right quantity. This saves time and should be fairly accurate.

Another tip I give my patients helps them cut down on salad dressing. I tell them to use a separate dish for the dressing and to dip each bite of salad into it, instead of pouring the dressing on the salad.

Gale Nunn, RN

Significant others

Preparing children for a parent's surgery

When my husband and I found out he was going to have open-heart surgery, we decided to prepare our young children for his stay in the hospital.

Before he was admitted, my husband videotaped himself reading bedtime stories. At the end of each story, he added his own message about what was probably happening to him each day. Each night he was hospitalized, I played one of the videos for our children.

I also put together a book of pictures they could color and send to him—one picture for each day. The pictures were posted in his room. Our children enjoyed this way of communicating with their dad, and they were less frightened about his surgery.

Luella Gillispie, RN, BSN

Rehab reinforcement

Here are two ways of reinforcing the benefits of rehabilitation:

When you help a patient with his morning care, make sure you use any adaptive equipment he's received from physical or occupational therapy. That way, he'll become familiar with the equipment, and he'll be more likely to use it when he's discharged.

If a patient has a therapy session during visiting hours, encourage family members to accompany him. This could help make discharge planning easier because family members will be more aware of the patient's limitations.

Linda G. Fuller, RN, BSN

Plastic stockings: Leg work

We try to provide hands-on teaching for the families of our cardiovascular patients. For example, the thigh-high elastic stockings that patients must wear for 1 month after discharge are hard to put on. We borrow an artificial leg from physical therapy and let family members practice putting the stockings on that.

Sherrie Holck, RN

Model for trach care

To teach a patient and his family members about tracheostomy care, hollow out a foam toy football. Place the inner cannula into this hollowed-out section, then tie the trach ties around the football. Doing this will give the patient and family members a feel for how the cannula should go in and come out. Allow them to take the model home so they can practice and teach other family members.

Cathy Farmer, RN,C

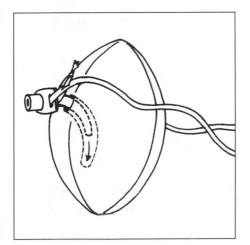

Table for teaching

The infant-care classes in our hospital nursery run more smoothly now that we have a special storage table. The table, built by our carpentry department, measures 30" x 58" x 36" and is enclosed in the front and on both sides. All items we use for class—such as bottles, diapers, dolls, a tub, handouts, notebooks, and pens—are neatly stored, and they're easily accessible from behind. Because it's on wheels, we can move the table if we need to arrange the classroom differently.

Florence Smith-Heney, RN

Teaching ventilation

If a baby on your unit has a tracheostomy and occasionally needs artificial ventilation when he becomes apneic and stimulation won't arouse him, you'll need to teach his mother how to ventilate him at home.

To help her practice, make a model respiratory system from the following materials: two finger cots, two rubber bands, a small Y-connector, some oxygen tubing, and a trach tube. Use the Y-connector to attach the finger cots to the oxygen tubing, securing them with the rubber bands. Then, attach the trach tube to the other end of the tubing. Finally, attach a hand-held resuscitation bag to the trach tube.

Now the mother can practice gauging the amount and rate of

pressure needed to inflate the finger-cot "lungs." When she becomes proficient in ventilating the model, she can take the baby home.

J. Thuman, RN

Think THUNDER

One of my pediatric patients had chronic otitis media. To teach his parents the signs and symptoms to watch for, I developed the acronym THUNDER. It stands for:

Temperature
Hearing loss
Upper respiratory infections
Nausea
Dizziness
Earache
Red ears.

I reminded the parents that otitis media feels like "thunder" in their child's ears, and I wrote the signs and symptoms on an index card for them to take home and keep as a reference.

Emoke Lukacs, SN

Say it with flowers

If you ever have to explain collateral circulation to a myocardial infarction patient and his family, compare your patient's injured vessel to the stem of a plant that's been accidentally broken off. When placed in a glass of water and given some time and care, the stem will sprout new roots. So, too, the patient's heart with proper care and rest will sprout new vessels.

Not only does this explanation bring a difficult subject into clearer focus, but it also gives the patient some much-needed hope for recovery.

Diana McLeod, RN

The public

Leading questions

I have many patient-teaching opportunities on our short-stay surgery unit. For example, when doing preoperative assessment of a pediatric patient, I might weigh the patient and say, making sure his parents are listening, "I see you weigh 33 pounds, Justin. You must still be riding in a car seat."

The parents usually respond to such a comment, giving me the chance to review local car-seat regulations.

Rose Coalson, RN, BSN

School sleuths

If you're a school nurse, teach the home economics and physical education teachers how to spot shoulder and hip disproportions—sewing classes and locker rooms are ideal places to spot scoliosis.

Sherry French, RN

More than just a "fair" idea

When 7-year-old Betsy went to the hospital to have her lacerated knee stitched, she impressed the nurses with her cooperation. Although

Betsy had never been to a hospital before, she knew a lot about it. Why? Because she was one of the thousands of children who attended the Bronson Young People's Health Fair, sponsored by the Bronson Methodist Hospital of Kalamazoo, Michigan.

Like Betsy, children usually come to the hospital only if they're ill or injured. But once a year, the hospital comes to them. Hospital personnel take their equipment to a city park; here, children ages 4 to 18 can learn about health care and safety. Nurses working at the fair involve the children through hands-on activities. For instance, one child stopped by the diabetes booth and told the nurse he was worried about his grandfather, who has diabetes. The nurse explained the disease to the child, telling him why his grandfather needed insulin injections. Then she had him inject "insulin" into an orange.

Nurses from all specialties work at the fair. An operating room nurse dressed in a scrub suit shows children instruments and anesthesia equipment. She explains what happens during a tonsillectomy and shows a storybook that illustrates the operation. Respiratory care nurses help children into a mist tent and give them balloons that demonstrate how the lungs work.

Children aren't the only ones who benefit from the fair. The hospital nurses appreciate the chance to meet with healthy children and to teach them how to stay healthy. The nurses also mingle with representatives from community service organizations, such as the public health department, the American Red Cross, and the child abuse council. This makes them more aware of referrals they can make when a patient is being discharged.

The nurses who have worked at the fairs say the event is always well received. Children leave with no-smoking buttons, cancer prevention comic books, and balloons. But even more important, they leave with a keener awareness of good health and a positive feeling about the hospital and the nurses who work there.

M.E. Martelli, RN;
A.M. Spaniolo, RN, MS;
B. Adams, RN

The staff

Round-the-clock education

Our hospital provides continuing education courses at all times of the day and night, so nurses on all shifts can take advantage of them. When we post notices of the courses, we include symbols—a sun, a setting sun, and the moon and stars for day, evening, and night, respectively—to indicate when each course is being offered. This way everyone can tell at a glance which courses are available to them.

Cheryl Arnett, RN
Cindy Rickel, RN

Teaching time

At the hospital where I work, we invite a staff doctor to speak on a topic of our choice at our monthly professional teaching rounds. These sessions are an excellent opportunity for us to discuss treatment rationales for specific cases and to improve nurse–doctor relations.

Debra A. Thompson, RN

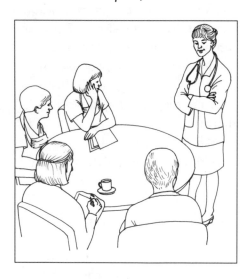

I.D.eal reference

In the emergency department where I work, we have to check and post laboratory results as we receive them. To remind myself of normal value ranges, I keep a list of them on an adhesive label on the back of my hospital identification card. This gives me a handy, helpful reference.

Diana Contine, RN

Quick reference guide

I work at a small hospital. Occasionally, we care for patients with unusual diagnoses. When this happens, I look up the condition in our unit's nursing reference books, then photocopy all pertinent information (including signs and symptoms, treatments, nursing considerations, and patient-teaching tips). I place this material in the patient's chart.

This way, any nurse caring for the patient can refer to the information. And when the patient is discharged, we can file it for future use.

Charles Dietzel, LPN

The answer album

To conserve space in our emergency department drug cabinet, we don't keep package inserts with the drugs in stock. Instead, we keep a photo album (the kind with clear, plastic pages) on top of the drug cabinet. In the plastic pages, we slip a package insert for each of the drugs we commonly use. When we have a question about one of these drugs, we just flip to that page in the album.

Kathleen Rohrer, RN

Drug of the month

I work in a newly opened recovery room with staff members from several different nursing backgrounds. To help us all become familiar with the many drugs used in the recovery room, we've initiated a "Drug of the Month" program.

Each month, one staff member researches a drug (such as Sublimaze or Innovar) and transcribes the fruits of her research onto a colorful, eye-catching poster. The poster is placed in the staff lounge or kitchen where nurses from all shifts can see it, read it, and learn.

Joanna P. Couch, RN, CCRN

Medication checklist

On our medication cart we keep a list, compiled by our hospital pharmacy, of commonly used drugs, including trade and generic names. If the pharmacy sends us a drug under a trade name we're not familiar with, we can check the list quickly to make sure we have the right drug.

Catherine H. Johnson, RN

Drugs in the news

The nurses at my hospital needed a handy source for the latest drug information. So the staff-development coordinator, a pharmacist, and I developed a newsletter—called *Medication Capsules*—that we distribute twice a month. The newsletter, only a half-page long, discusses new drugs, pertinent drug topics derived from medication errors, questions from staff nurses, and incident reports. We stick to the facts nurses need to know. We post current newsletters on each medication cart and file old ones in the back of the Kardex.

Kathleen Ellstrom, RN, CCRN, MS

Ready reference

We've developed a handy reference that staff nurses can carry in their pockets. On 2" x 3" index cards, we write reference information about lab values, I.V. calculations, nursing diagnoses, and so on. We laminate each card, punch a hole in one end, then place the cards on a key ring. We keep the ring at the nurses' station.

The reference cards started out as a unit project, but as other units heard about it, they decided to contribute. We now have cards from the intensive care unit, the operating room, and the post-anesthesia room.

Kathy Baskin, RN
Gerri Danto, RN

Keeping new information handy

If you're just graduating, changing clinical areas, or reentering nursing, here's a tip for you.

Buy 3" x 5" index cards and a ring binder notebook designed to hold them. Each time you learn something new (such as a procedure or a handy tip), write it on a card and snap the card into your book.

My book includes drawings of machines and how to use them, drug-incompatibility lists, and a few phonetically written words in several foreign languages.

R.W. Keyser-McClendon, RN

What nerves

When I was in nursing school, I devised this number drawing to help me remember the 12 cranial nerves.

Beneath the drawing, I listed the nerves that correspond with the numbers in the picture. Then I named some of the actions or sensations controlled by those nerves. My list looked like this:

1. *Olfactory*—smell
2. *Optic*—vision

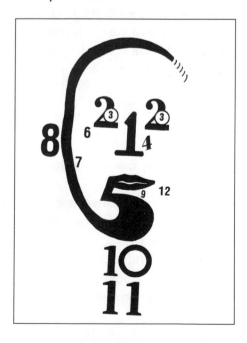

3. *Oculometer*—iris and eye movements
4. *Trochlear*—eye movements
5. *Trigeminal*—upper and lower mouth and teeth, forehead, anterior half of scalp
6. *Abducens*—eye movement (lateral)
7. *Facial*—facial expression
8. *Acoustic*—hearing, balance
9. *Glossopharyngeal*—tastebuds on posterior part of tongue, throat sensations, saliva secretions
10. *Vagus*—swallowing, vocal cords, goes to abdominal organs
11. *Accessory*—head and shoulder movements
12. *Hypoglossal*—chewing, speaking, swallowing.

The drawing was a handy study aid in school, and it's a handy reference now.

Beatrice Humphris, RN

Photo opportunity

Here's how to help the staff become more familiar with what's in a code cart. Photograph the contents of each drawer (in color) and paste the photos on a large sheet of poster board. Label each picture with its corresponding drawer. Then hang the poster on a wall where everyone can see it.

Edwina A. McConnell, RN, PhD

Teaching tape

When a quadriplegic patient is transferred from our rehabilitation hospital to a nursing home, we send along a videotape showing one of our nurses taking care of the patient. The tape helps the nurses at the nursing home understand what needs to be done for the patient. Our nurses explain special procedures and techniques and possible complications related to the patient's care—good practice in strengthening their teaching skills.

If possible, the patient participates in the teaching process, too, by pointing out aspects of his care that are particularly beneficial.

Pat Houdart, RN

In the cards

When caring for ostomy patients, we put "appliance cards" in each patient's Kardex. The cards describe the proper procedure for changing the patient's appliance. They also note the date of each appliance change and list order numbers for various supplies.

Jill Conwill, RN, ET

Insulin in order

As you draw up fast-acting and long-lasting insulins into the same syringe, remember this phrase to get the order right: *Fast first, long last.*

Maureen Anthony, RN

Fractions of 60

To help calculate the flow rate of I.V. fluids, I teach my students the "Fractions of 60." If an I.V. set delivers 60 drops/ml, the drops/minute rate equals the number of milliliters delivered in 1 hour. For sets delivering a fraction of 60 drops/ml, use the formula below, based on administering 120 ml/hour, to determine the drops/minute:

Set delivers	Fraction of 60	Drops/ minute
60 drops/ml	1: (120÷1)	120
20 drops/ml	1/3: (120÷3)	40
15 drops/ml	1/4: (120÷4)	30
10 drops/ml	1/6: (120÷6)	20

With this formula, your students won't need pencil and paper to figure out I.V. flow rates.

Sue Wisenbaker, RN, MA

Practice shots

Injecting needles into an orange doesn't give student nurses the feel of tissue penetration that accompanies real injections. Try letting them practice on uncooked chicken breasts with the skin still attached. Using a realistic model like that can better prepare them for the real thing.

Amy Swango, RN, MSN

Learning about burns

As a clinical instructor for a regional burn unit, I teach nurses how to debride blistered, burned skin. To do this, I give the nurses plastic sheets of packing bubbles. Then I show them how to puncture the bubbles and cut away the plastic, using the same instruments and techniques they'll use to debride real skin.

Lori Jurgens, RN, CCRN

Pillow practice

Ever since I designed a special pillow "abdomen," my students get lots of practice in advancing Penrose drains and removing sutures. If these procedures are included in your state's nurse practice act, you might want to try this idea, too.

To make an abdomen, I cover a pillow-sized, foam-rubber square with about 36" of heavy, skin-colored, synthetic suede material. When sewing the seam, I leave a 2" to 3" gap along one side. This allows me to replace the Penrose drain periodically.

On one face of the pillow, to the left side, I make a small slit through which the Penrose drain will protrude, to mimic a drain protruding from a patient's incision. To the right of this (or anywhere you wish), I make a long slit—or "surgical incision"—and sew it together with silk sutures. And for atmosphere, I add a belly button.

As students advance the Penrose drain through the small slit, the foam inside the abdomen offers a slight resistance, simulating actual drain advancement. Practicing this procedure and having the chance to repeatedly remove sutures helps give the students the confidence they'll need when they do the real thing.

Kay Segundo, RN

Interpreting tricky rhythms

Occasionally, even the most experienced nurses on our telemetry unit have trouble analyzing a cardiac rhythm strip. We've started keeping problematic strips in a book that we call "Name That Rhythm." During slow periods on the unit, we help each other interpret the rhythms.

Linda Tate, RN, BSN

Readin', writin', and arrhythmias

I work in a small 4-bed ICU where we don't see many life-threatening arrhythmias. To be sure the staff will be able to recognize an arrhythmia when it occurs, about every 2 weeks I give each person a sheet of rhythm strips to study. Later we review the strips together. The staff finds the sessions helpful—especially when the next life-threatening arrhythmia actually does occur.

Margery Lebel, RN, CCRN

Poster prop

At the small hospital where I work, we use large posters as reminders during a code. We use a black felt-tip pen and cardboard from X-ray film to make a set of easy-to-read posters, and we keep them right where we need them—on the crash cart.

On each poster, we put one procedure used during a code, such as defibrillation. Whoever is the recorder during the code selects and sets up the appropriate poster as needed.

Barbara Schoonover, RN

Picture this

At the nursing home where I work, some of the residents who use a wheelchair have adaptive devices (braces, arm holders, and so forth) to keep them properly positioned and supported. To make sure that all staff members know how to use these devices, we take photographs of the residents from several angles, showing them correctly outfitted. We mount the photos on paper, label them with instructions, then hang the photos on the inside of the residents' bedside cabinets.

Nancy Harrold, RN

See how they grow

To teach staff members the importance of infection-control practices, have them conduct a clinical experiment: making their own cultures to see how quickly bacteria grow.

First, get four agar plates. Then have the staff take cultures from their hands, the bottoms of their shoes, a bedside stand, and a patient's overbed table—especially one who places used tissues on the table rather than discarding them After taking the cultures and labeling the plates, take them to the laboratory to be incubated for 48 hours.

Later, share the report from the laboratory. The results will show the nursing staff the importance of maintaining cleanliness.

Cherry A. Karl, RN, BSN

3 ADULT PATIENT CARE

Fluid and nutrition

Color their world

If your sight-impaired patient has trouble getting food onto his fork, use colored dishes and bowls so he can see his food more easily. I've found that dark colors such as black, green, and blue are most helpful, especially for patients who have bilateral macular degeneration or cataracts.

Marilla E. Petersen, RN, MS

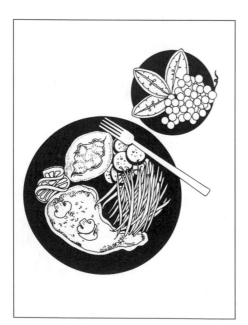

Simple snack

Here's a tasty and nutritious snack you can make for patients with poor appetites. Slice or mash a banana, then mix it up with sugar and whole milk. For diabetic patients, use a sugar substitute and skim milk.

Lucy M. Wasowski, RN

A good shake

When a patient wants—and *needs*—a high-calorie, high-protein bedtime snack but the hospital's kitchen is closed, what can you do? Take a look at the snacks stored in your unit's refrigerator and improvise.

For example, you can mix a carton or two of any flavor of ice cream with milk for a quick, nutritious, and appetizing milk shake. (Let the ice cream soften slightly first for easier mixing.) Or mix some sherbet with a liquid elemental diet, such as Vivonex. Patients will like these shakes—and benefit from their nutritional value too.

Vicki Ephrou, RN

Lip service

A great gift idea for a patient who can't eat or drink anything is an assortment of different-flavored lip balms. The pleasant taste of the lip balm will help satisfy the patient's craving for flavor, while the moisturizing emollients will help soothe his parched, cracked lips.

Paula Brenton, RN

Decarbonation

For a patient who needs fluids and would like to have a soda but can't tolerate its carbonation, try stirring about ¼ teaspoon sugar into the soda. The sugar will neutralize the carbonation. Patients who've had throat surgery or radiation therapy, as well as ulcer patients, will appreciate this tip.

Judith Snow, RN, CMS

More pleasing by freezing

When a patient has trouble swallowing because of throat surgery or a hampered gag reflex resulting from a stroke, taking liquids may be a problem. But freezing liquids is helpful. Patients can swallow high-protein and high-calorie items such as Sustacal, milk shakes, and eggnog much more easily when they're in a semi-solid state. Another advantage: freezing makes less desirable liquids more palatable.

Barbara D. Mizenko, RN

Ice pop therapy

When you need to increase a patient's oral fluid intake, try giving him homemade flavored ice pops. Here's my recipe:

First, fill plastic medication cups about three-quarters full with juice. Freeze them until they turn to slush, then insert a coffee stirrer in each. Then freeze them until they're solid.

Paula Mininger, RN

Juicy way to stretch fluids

I make juice cubes by freezing several kinds of fruit juices in 15-ml medication cups. This adds variety to a fluid-restricted diet and makes the fluid allotment last.

Kathleen A. Janka, RN, BSN

Soup's on

During my evening rounds, I offer my patients a snack, if orders allow. Because the hospital usually serves cold, boxed snacks at this time of the day, I try to offer the patient something hot as well. Serving a hot drink or chicken soup mix that requires only hot water is no trouble at all and frequently satisfies my patients.

Betty Francis, LPN

The pop that refreshes

Patients on fluid restrictions have thirsts to satisfy, like anyone else. But small quantities of liquids that get swallowed in one sip aren't very satisfying.

To quench patients' thirsts and still keep accurate intake/output records, make flavored ice pops from juice or an allowed supplement. Pour the liquid into 30-ml cups, insert an orangewood stick in each, and then put the cups in the freezer. When you're ready to use the ice pops, loosen the cups by running them under warm water for a few seconds. Patients really enjoy these treats, and they stay within their fluid limits.

Mary Massaro, RN

Spray thirst away

Do you have patients on restricted fluid intake? You can help them quench their thirst while using only a small amount of their allotted liquid by using a plastic squeeze bottle with a spray top.

Here's how. At the beginning of your shift, check to see what the patient's allotted amount of fluid is. For example, if he's allowed 50 ml of fluid during the shift, he may wish to use half his allotment in the water spray bottle. Then fill the bottle with 25 ml of water and let the patient spray his mouth as he feels the need. At the end of your shift, measure the remaining amount of water in the bottle. If, for instance, it is 5 ml, you would record an intake of 20 ml from the spray bottle, plus whatever other fluid intake he's had during your shift.

Chris Christgau, RN

Short straw

When patients are weak but need to take fluids by mouth, I cut off a piece of straw about 3" long and let them drink through it. They don't expend as much energy drinking through this shortened straw.

Mary J. Muzyczyn, RN, BSN

Put a lid on it

Some bedridden patients spill more than they drink whenever they use a cup or glass. So ask their families to bring in an empty pint-size jar with a screw-on lid. (A mayonnaise jar is a good example.)

With a nail that has about the same diameter as a straw, punch a hole in the middle of the lid. Then pour the liquid into the jar, screw on the lid, and put a straw through the hole. The patient can drink away—and not spill anymore.

Deann Meyers, RN

Drink up: Handy bottle for fluids

A plastic squeeze bottle with a built-in straw works well for a patient who has to drink a lot of fluid. It also helps to eliminate bedside clutter because he won't need so many cups for juice and water.

Each bottle holds about 32 oz of fluid. If you need precise input and output measurements, place a piece of tape on the side of the bottle and label it appropriately (in ounces or milliliters).

These bottles are inexpensive and can be purchased at any convenience store. And they're easy to clean with soap and water.

Pat White, RN

When it pumps, it pours

Some of our patients lack the strength and coordination to pour water or juice from a pitcher into a cup. To make sure they get their required fluids, we give each of them a "pump pot"—a small picnic jug with a spout that dispenses liquid when you push down on the lid.

Usually, patients can fill their cups themselves with the pump pots, so they're encouraged to take more fluids. We like the pots, too: they save us the time of refilling cups. And since they're insulated, we don't have to refill the pots with ice.

Jeanne Sorrell, RN

Pick from the bucket

Here's a way to encourage fluid intake for a patient who's ordered to "force fluids up to 3 liters/day." Ask the food service department to send up a plastic bucket (one for each shift) filled with ice and eight 4-oz plastic cups. Fill the cups with at least four different kinds of juice and cap with spillproof lids.

Leave the bucket at the patient's bedside. The patient will look forward to choosing his next drink from his juice bucket. With this reminder, you won't have to remind

him to take his fluids.

Jane S. McDermott, RN, BS

Watermelon magic

When a patient's treatment includes forcing fluids, do you find *yourself* doing the forcing? Solve the fluid problem (at least in the summer months) by serving watermelon. The fruit is loaded with water, it's cold and nutritious, and patients love it!

Barbara Neale, RN

Mixed drinks

To help your patient comply with his orders to drink a lot of fluids, try this: fill his plastic washbasin with some ice and several cans or cartons of his favorite juices or sodas. Place the basin at the patient's bedside, where he can reach it easily.

The patient will appreciate having a variety of fluids other than water on hand, and he'll be more likely to comply with orders to "drink up."

Claire E. Mendenhall, RN

Gripping solution

Many patients with arthritis in their hands have trouble gripping eating utensils, pens, and pencils. To enlarge the grip on these and other slender items, use foam cylinders from hair curlers. A package of about 10 costs approximately $1, and they're avail-

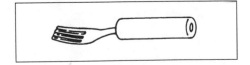

able in many drug and department stores. Just slip the foam cylinder off the plastic curler spindle and onto the slender pen or handle.

Evelyn Rossky, OT

Gripping idea

For a patient who doesn't have full use of his hands, try placing a terry cloth wristband around his drinking container. The wristband will allow the patient to grip the container more easily by himself, which should help him to feel more independent.

Pat O'Donnell, LPN

Rubber grip for cups

Here's an easy solution for a patient who has trouble grasping his cup or the handle of his mug.

Wrap three rubber bands around the cup or mug's handle. (You can also use them on the pitcher's handle.) Now your patient will have something to grip.

Rubber bands are inexpensive and easy to find. When your patient goes home, you can even send a handful of them with him.

Terrilynn M. Quillen, RN

Getting a grip on utensils

When a stroke patient has difficulty grasping silverware, try wrapping Velcro strips around the knife, fork, and spoon handles. The patient will find it easier to grip the handles.

Peggy Giaimo, RN

Spoons for the elderly

To feed an elderly patient, try using a small, plastic-coated spoon (the kind used for babies). The spoon holds a more manageable portion that's easier to swallow. Plus, the soft coating is less irritating to sensitive gums.

B. Felker, RN

Cup of encouragement

An elderly patient had trouble drinking out of a regular glass and refused to drink through a straw. So I asked his family to bring in a plastic cup with a sipper lid. Because the patient was able to use this cup without spills, he could drink the required amount of fluid each day.

Vicki L. Miller, LPN

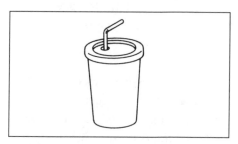

Staying in control

Even if he's using a straw, a patient may have trouble drinking from a cup. A training cup may solve the problem. These cups have handles on both sides and a lid on top, so the patient can drink by himself and still have some control. And if he drops it, he won't make much of a mess.

Sandra McIntosh, LPN

Stationary dishes

A patient with upper arm weakness may have a problem with dishes sliding around on his tray. So I put a rubber bottle-cap opener under each dish. (The openers are available at hardware stores and housewares departments of discount department stores.) This holds the dishes in place so the patient can eat with less difficulty.

Bonnie Faherty, RN, CS

Pad for soaking up spills

If a patient has difficulty feeding himself, he may end up spilling his meal. Here's an easy way to protect his gown.

Place a disposable blue pad over the front of the patient, with the absorbent side facing out to soak up spills. Use a piece of tape to anchor each side of the pad to the patient's gown at his shoulders. You can also form a pocket at the bottom of the pad to prevent large pieces of food, such as vegetables, from falling onto the floor. To do this, fold up 4" to 6" of the pad and tape the sides together.

The patient won't soil himself or his bed—and you'll avoid extra linen changes.

Sonja Jones, RN

Apron catchall

A full-length vinyl chef's apron works well for a stroke patient who's learning to feed himself again. It catches spills, and it's more dignified than a geriatric bib. These inexpensive aprons come in a variety of colors and styles.

Terrilynn M. Quillen, RN

Mobility

Lights on

When a patient has trouble turning on his overhead light, a piece of elastic gauze may help. Cut a long, narrow strip of the gauze. Then, tie one end to the light cord and the other end to the upper side rail of the patient's bed. The patient will be able to turn the light on and off by himself. For a brighter touch, try using a single stitch crochet chain made from colored yarn.

Lynn Boggio, RN

Smooth move

When I need to transfer an obese patient from one bed to another, I slide the patient *and* his mattress onto the new bed. Mattress handles make this easy to accomplish. This method reduces strain and discomfort for both the patient and nurse. It also works well with patients who have difficulty moving.

Fay Stout, RN

Rehab roll

In the rehabilitation hospital where I work, we encourage patients with total hip replacements to propel their own wheelchairs. But most patients have trouble with this because they're too busy trying to keep the abduction pillow between their knees.

We solved the problem by making an abduction pillow that stays in place. We wrap adhesive tape around a rolled towel (so it stays rolled up) and tie long pieces of gauze to the tape. Then we tie the ends of the gauze to the wheelchair.

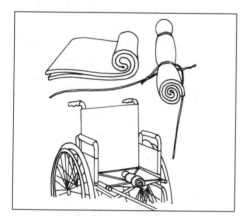

Now the patient can propel his wheelchair and not worry that the towel will slide out from between his knees.

Victoria A. Schnaufer, LPN

A good move for mobility

When patients need to improve mobility in their shoulders and arms, recommend effective exercises that are fun, too. Recently, I had some transient paralysis on the right side of my body from a stroke. My favorite exercise was practicing basketball shots with a soft foam ball and a hoop. The toy was inexpensive and easy to set up. The shooting movement improved the range of motion in my right shoulder and arm.

Kathleen Lissenden, RN

Walking: Count on it

When my father developed Parkinson's disease, the hardest part of walking for him was getting started. His neurologist recommended walking to a march-style beat (*one-two-three-four, one-two-three-four*), which I would say out loud. I recorded several minutes of this counting rhythm on a small tape recorder, which my father carries in his pocket. Now he can start walking on his own simply by turning on the tape.

Arlene Evans, RN, PHN

Hook the bag

Have trouble ambulating a patient who has an indwelling catheter by yourself? Ask the hospital maintenance department to put a hook on the lower part of each movable I.V. pole. This hook holds the catheter bag more securely than a pin on the patient's clothing. Also, the patient can hold on to the I.V. pole for stability—and you can ambulate him by yourself.

One caution: Make sure the catheter tubing doesn't hang low between the patient and pole. Otherwise, the tubing could get caught under the pole's wheels.

Charlene Forvery, LPN

Gifts for the elderly

Volunteers at the nursing home where I work make items that our elderly residents can use every day.

For residents who have walkers or wheelchairs and for those who are bedridden, our volunteers make sturdy cloth bags. These bags have straps that button and pockets that can hold personal items, such as pens, combs, and tissues. The residents attach these bags to their walkers, wheelchairs, or bed rails. The volunteers also make decorative cloth covers for indwelling urinary catheter bags. These covers have drawstrings at the top so the bags can be removed easily.

Carolyn Cave, RN

Inside pocket

Ambulating patients with a Hemovac can be a problem. The solution? A secret inside pocket.

Pin a washcloth to the inside of the patient's robe to form a pocket. Then tell the patient to *drop* (not pin) the Hemovac into the pocket when he gets out of bed. This way, the Hemovac is out of sight and safe from being pulled out.

Linda Mitchell, RN

Supportive shoes

You can reduce foot drop in bedridden or immobilized patients by putting high-top sneakers on their feet during the day. For best results, make sure the laces are tied tightly.

Patti Moore, RN

One size fits all

Custom-fit disposable sponge slippers to a patient's foot size. Just tie a rubber band around the excess sponge at the slipper's heel, and it fits perfectly.

Peggy Young, RN, BSN

Nonslip slippers

Shiny hospital corridors can be hazardous to unsteady, recently postoperative or elderly patients. To help keep them from skidding—and boost their self-confidence—attach skidproof bathtub appliqués to the soles of their slippers. Or you can put stockinettes on the patient's feet and attach the appliqués to the bottoms.

To reinforce the appliqués so they'll withstand several washings, sew all around the edges.

And here's an even more economical tip—buy sheets of rubber that have an adhesive backing and cut out your own appliqués.

Ellen Roben, RN

Skidproof shoes

For the stroke patient who is just becoming ambulatory, firm, laced shoes with crepe or rubber soles are recommended. But if the patient doesn't have such shoes, you can make his own leather-soled tie shoes skidproof. Just fit a pair of foam rubber hospital slippers over the patient's shoes and anchor them with adhesive tape. This will provide both the support and the friction the patient needs to keep from slipping or sliding.

Renee Berke, RN

Foot cover-up

After we've finished dressing a patient's foot in the emergency department (ED), we protect it with a shoe cover similar to the ones used in the operating room. This helps keep the patient's foot warm and the dressing clean and dry. And he doesn't have to wear a shoe when he leaves the ED, eliminating the excess pressure a shoe would cause.

C.J. DeSantis, RN

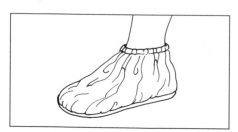

Restraints

Hands off

To prevent an elderly patient from pulling out his feeding tube or catheter without using wrist restraints, which restrict mobility, try this technique.

With the patient's fingers extended, wrap a piece of soft cloth around each hand. Then take two small inflatable tubes (the kind used on children's arms for swimming) and slide them onto the patient's hands. This prevents the patient from being able to manipulate his fingers. As a bonus, the tubes can help prevent contractures by maintaining good hand position.

Nancy J. Augustine, RN

Strapped no more

Soft strap restraints used to keep patients from pulling out their I.V.s, nasogastric tubes, and indwelling urinary catheters don't always work well. Some patients wiggle free of the restraints; others get confused and agitated because their movements are restricted. Sometimes the restraints even inhibit circulation to the patient's fingers.

Instead of straps, pull a stockinette over the patient's hand and up his arm as if it were a sleeve. Then secure the stockinette bottom around the patient's wrist with adhesive tape, being careful not to tape too tightly.

Next, put a sponge ball (the soft kind children play with) into the patient's hand, pull the stockinette back down his arm and over his taped wrist and hand, and tie a knot in the stockinette close to his fingers. Finally, repeat the procedure for the patient's other hand.

With both hands filled, the patient can't get hold of the I.V.s and other tubes. Still, he has freedom of movement—and he can squeeze the balls to exercise his fingers.

Kimberlee A. Hull, CVN

Vested wanderers

To keep track of confused patients who might wander off our unit, we give them lightweight, bright orange vests to wear when they leave their rooms. We've informed other units of this policy. So if one of our patients turns up on another unit, someone can always lead him back.

Jean Jordan, RN,C

Give 'em a boot

Give your patients with temporary transvenous pacemakers a boot—a Buck's traction boot, that is.

Simply place the patient's arm and the pulse generator in the boot, and fasten the straps to keep the arm immobile. If the patient's arm is longer than the boot, cut open the end of the boot. And, with confused patients, tie the boot to the bed with the attached traction rope. The boot's metal strip keeps the arm straight but less rigid than it would be with a conventional arm board. Also, the pulse generator can be kept alongside rather than on top of the arm, adding to patient comfort.

Keep a Buck's traction boot on your pacemaker cart, because it's just the boot some patients need.

Joan Belisle, RN

Physical care

Glow-in-the-dark clipboard

I put reflector tape on the bedside clipboards so I can easily spot them at night. This saves me from blindly searching a patient's room in the dark and possibly disturbing him. Glow-in-the-dark stickers work just as well.

Kathryn Kilcrease, RN

Cloth case for eyeglasses

When a hospitalized patient forgets to bring a case for his glasses, I make one for him. I fold a washcloth in half, then in thirds. I tape the flap shut, and write the patient's name on the tape. Then I close one of the open ends with another piece of tape.

Lillian C. Tieman, RN

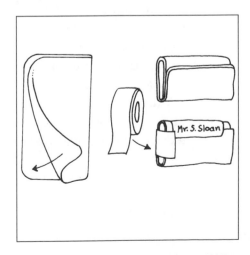

Blue dots for diabetic patients

I work in a doctor's office. To identify a diabetic patient quickly, I place a large blue dot on the bottom of his chart. When I pull the chart before the patient's appointment, I'm reminded that I'll need to allow time to test his blood glucose level; review his weight, diet, and medications; and examine his feet.

Marlu Eisner, RN

Hearty tip

To keep transducers for central venous and pulmonary artery catheters at the level of the patient's heart, I use an electrode patch. I remove the pad's adhesive, except for the small tab, secure the pad at the appropriate level, and clip the transducer to the tab. This works especially well for diaphoretic patients.

Ruth Brye-Braden, RN, CCRN, BSN

Breathing to the beat

When a patient is being weaned from a ventilator, he can easily become panicked—which will accelerate his respirations. To solve this problem, we've started to use a metronome—a device musicians use to mark time while they're playing. It can be set at different rates to mimic the desired breathing pattern. The regular ticking calms the patient and allows him to focus on slower, fuller breathing.

Patti Acton, RN, BSN

Oximeter probe cover

I've found that a finger cot placed over a disposable oximeter probe can prolong the probe's usefulness. The cot discourages the patient from picking at tape edges, prevents the edges from catching on linens, and may also allow probe use after the tape has lost some adherence.

Ann Andel, RN, BSN

Tab your tape

Here's a fast, easy way to remove tape from a patient's skin. After applying the tape, fold up one of the corners, leaving a small tab. Now you have something to grab when you want to remove the tape—and you won't have to dig into the patient's skin.

And to eliminate extra discomfort, rub the patient's skin with alcohol or water to help dissolve the adhesive that's left behind.

Annette Bryant, RN

DuoDERM dressing: Covered and clean

When an incontinent patient needs a DuoDERM dressing on an area that can get soiled, I cover the DuoDERM with a clean TEgaderm. That way, I can remove the tegaderm as needed and replace it with a new one—without having to disturb the DuoDERM.

Nancy Redner, RN

Cotton convenience

To absorb perspiration and moisture under a patient's natural body folds (such as under the breasts), I use cotton batting, which comes on a roll. This works especially well if a patient has irritated skin—I just apply powder to the area and then place a strip of the cotton under the fold. The cotton prevents the powder from caking and is less cumbersome than gauze pads.

Carole Oberle, RN, CETN, MSN

Clever cover

I devised a good way to cover a gauze dressing on an arm or leg wound. Just cut off the reinforced top of a knee-high stocking and slip it over the dressing. The cover is cool, it's easy to apply, and it fits snugly without tape. The elastic band can be washed, dried, and reused. And its skin-tone color makes the dressing less noticeable.

Cheryl Moose, RN

Bedside baskets

For a patient who requires frequent dressing changes, we keep all the necessary supplies in a wire basket by his bed. We restock the basket every day.

Amor Gonzales-Carethers, RN,C

Innovative eye patch

I once cared for a patient with a painful nasopharyngeal cancer who needed to wear an eye patch overnight. However, our supply department didn't have an eye patch that I could secure with an elastic band—and the patient couldn't tolerate a hard plastic patch taped to his head.

So I detached the oxygen connector tube from a tracheostomy collar and placed four round gauze pads over his eye. Then I put the mask over his eye and secured it around his head with the mask's elastic band.

The mask held the gauze pads in place and didn't cause any additional pain for the patient.

Janine M. Seipel-Lattuca, RN

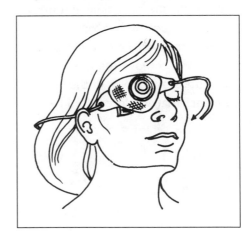

Impromptu colostomy collection

Here's what I do when a colostomy patient with diarrhea is admitted to our unit at night.

I open the end of the drainable colostomy pouch, slip ½ of a large-lumen rectal tube into it, then secure the tube and pouch with two rubber bands. I attach the other end of the rectal tube to tubing on a closed drainage collection bag and hang the bag over the side of the bed.

The watery stool drains into the bag, so I don't have to disturb the patient to empty the colostomy pouch frequently. I still get an accurate output measurement, and the patient can get a good night's rest without being bothered.

S. Simon, RN, BSN

Colostomy bag: Cuff and clean

Try this tip the next time you need to empty a colostomy bag:

Hold the bottom of the bag up slightly and remove the clip. Roll the clean bottom portion of the bag (the part that was protected by the

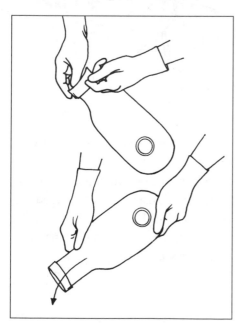

clip) over like the cuff on a pant leg. Then lower the bag, remove the contents, and clean the inside. Finally, roll the clean cuff down and reapply the clip.

This simple procedure keeps the bottom of the colostomy bag clean and free from odor.

Anne Marie Ferris, RN

Oiling the ostomy pouch

I always smear drops of vegetable oil inside an ostomy pouch before using it. Then when I'm ready to empty the pouch, the contents slide out easily and nothing sticks to the sides. This reduces unnecessary pouch changes and costs incurred by the patient and facility.

Kathy Ptacin, RN

Colostomy wafer: Tracing the perfect fit

When caring for a patient with a colostomy, I've found that the stoma isn't always exactly round, like the colostomy wafer. So I place a piece of clear plastic wrap against the stoma and trace it with a marker. Then I use the outline as my pattern for cutting the wafer. This way, the wafer will fit perfectly around the stoma.

Barbara Ann Gonzalez, RN

Cut and dry

I cut a ¼" to ⅜" slit at the top and bottom center of the adhesive portion of fecal incontinence bags. The

bag adheres more evenly to the patient and it's less likely to leak.
Angelina Elkin, RN

Keeping a catheter in place
The skin cement or bond that's used with colostomy supplies also keeps external catheters in place. It's more effective than tape or tincture of benzoin, and it doesn't irritate the patient's skin.
Laurie Ellsworth, RN

Trach cover-up
We tie a surgical mask around a tracheostomy patient's neck when he wants to leave his bed. The mask keeps foreign objects out of the trach, protects staff and other patients from projectile sputum, and allows us to check secretions. And because the trach is covered, the patient is less self-conscious.
Michelle Kopinski, LPN

Bedpan plan
For a female patient who has difficulty getting on and off a bedpan, I use a disposable emesis basin. Hold the basin gently against the patient's perineum while she urinates. Always have a second basin ready in case one isn't enough to hold her urine.

I find this method especially helpful for female patients with fractured hips.
Victoria Burke, RN, BSN

Powdered bedpan
Here's a way to help a patient who has to use a bedpan. Sprinkle some powder around the top of the rim so that the bedpan slides underneath the patient more easily.
Margaret Farny, RN

Dry linens
For male patients who wet their bed linen when using urinals, try this idea. Cut a hole in the center of a disposable underpad and place it, absorbent side up, over the patient's urinal. Instruct the patient to put his penis through the hole when urinating. This keeps the bed clean and dry and prevents an embarrassing situation for the patient.
Mary Moriarty Villani, BSN
Margie White, LPN

Securing stockings
The antiembolism stockings we use under pneumatic compression devices typically roll at the top, forming a tourniquet around the patient's thigh. To prevent this, we fold the stocking over the top of the pneumatic compression device cuff. This prevents stricture and is more comfortable for the patient.
Laureen Koontzy, LVN

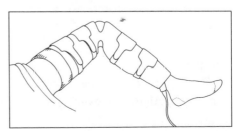

Covering
Do you use surgical tape to secure a patient's ring to his finger before surgery? If so, do you find a sticky, hard-to-remove film on the ring's stone when you take the tape off?

Next time, use an adhesive bandage (with the gauze pad over the stone) to secure the ring. When you remove the bandage, the stone's beauty will be unblemished.

N. May, RN

In the pot
We keep a ready supply of warm, moist towels in a slow-cooker, set on low. (Our engineering department modified the plug for safety.) The towels come in handy for breast-feeding mothers. They can also be used to dilate veins before starting I.V.s.

Lucinda Powers, RN, BSN

Creative compress
The next time you need a hot, moist compress, try using a disposable diaper. Soak the diaper in water, then heat it in a microwave oven, set on "high," for 45 seconds. Check to make sure it's not too hot, then apply it to the site. The diaper will retain heat and moisture longer than most compresses.

Robin Jones, RN

Ice pack
Here's a good way to make ice packs for patients recovering from tooth extractions. Take a gallon-size plastic bag (the kind that "zips" closed), fill it with a few ice cubes and water, and put it in a pillowcase to absorb moisture. The pack will fit nicely on the patient's jaw and will stay in place while he sleeps.

Jill Dailer, RN, BSN

Nice ice
To make ice bags that aren't too hard, add some rubbing alcohol to the water before freezing it. The result will be a firm slush, easy for the patient to hold.

Phyllis Henning, RN, BSN, MN

Keeping ice packs in place
After oral or facial surgery, many of the patients on our postanesthesia care unit need ice packs. But we had trouble keeping those packs in place. Here's how I solved the problem.

I cut a 3' piece of 3" wide orthopedic stockinette. After tying a knot in the center, I insert an ice pack in one or both ends, depending on the type of surgery the patient had. Then I tie the stockinette at the top of the patient's head, with the knot under his chin.

The ice pack remains in place without slipping. And the patient is comfortable.

Mark Peplow, RN

Postop reminder cards
With the help of our physical thera-

pists, we developed "recovery cards" to remind us of positioning and activity restrictions for postoperative orthopedic patients. The appropriate card is placed in a plastic folder and left at the head of the patient's bed.

Besides being great reminders for us, the cards also help float nurses, agency nurses, and nursing students who may not be familiar with orthopedic patients and the restrictions necessary for recovery.

Mary Jemmett, RN

Laceration lubrication

If a scalp laceration is hard to suture because the patient's hair gets entangled in the suture material (even though the wound area has been prepared), try this technique. After you've shaved the area, apply a sterile, water-soluble lubricant around the hairline of the laceration. This will hold the hair down, preventing it from getting entangled in the suture and providing a more sterile field. The lubricant can be easily washed out after suturing.

Linda Drain, RN
Cheryl Westbay, RN

A clear chaser

To hasten vomiting after administering a dose of ipecac syrup, offer the patient a clear soft drink such as ginger ale or 7-Up. The soft drink is more palatable than the warm water that's usually given, and its carbonation makes the patient feel full. A word of caution, though: The soft drink produces results quickly—so be prepared.

Grace Redheffer, RN, BSN

Filter cap for pigtail port

I've found an easy solution to a draining pigtail port on a Salem sump tube. I save the air-permeable, water-resistant filter caps that come on some types of I.V. tubing. After I set up an I.V. line, I insert a cap in the pigtail port of the Salem sump tube as needed. The cap allows air to pass into the pigtail while preventing fluid reflux. When the cap becomes soiled, I simply replace it.

The cap keeps gowns and bed linens from becoming soiled by refluxed gastric contents, and I don't have to spend time changing linens.

Anita J. Rider, RN

Comfortable fit

A patient with a nasogastric (NG) tube and an oxygen face mask may be uncomfortable if the mask presses on the tube. You can solve this by cutting a small slit on the top of the face mask. Make sure you have a good seal on the mask. Place the mask under the NG tube so the tube rests on top of it. They fit together well, and your patient will be more comfortable.

Sara Sloan, RN

Keeping a nasal cannula in place

At our long-term care facility, we encourage a patient who's receiving oxygen through a nasal cannula to leave his eyeglasses on. The glasses will keep the tubing taut and hold the cannula snugly in place without blocking airflow.

Pat White, RN

Shoe cover: Fit for a foot

If a patient is discharged from our emergency department with a dressing that prevents him from putting on his shoe, I give him a disposable shoe cover to wear instead. This way, the dressing stays clean.

Phoebe Hershenow, RN, BSN

Colorful system for identifying tests

Many of our psychiatric patients require laboratory tests or other diagnostic procedures. But if a patient cannot or will not cooperate, the tests or procedures may be delayed; the staff needs a way to know that other than by checking the patient's Kardex.

To solve the problem, we developed a color-coded dot system, using ¾" stickers for specific tests or procedures. For example, red is for urine toxicology; gold, for 24-hour urine specimens; black, for chest X-rays; and so on. We place the appropriate stickers on a piece of paper, then slip the paper into the name holder outside a patient's door. As each test or procedure is completed, we remove the dots.

Joan C. Masters, RN, MA
Susan F. Barati, MHT

Armboard pad: A quick cushion

Here's a quick way to pad an armboard: Position a small disposable diaper—plastic side down—on the armboard, then tape it in place.

Anne Knapp, RN

Stretcher point

When an ED patient's condition allows it, I use what I call a modified Trendelenburg position to make him more comfortable on a stretcher. I raise the head and the foot of the stretcher about 20 degrees each. Then I place a pillow under the patient's knees. This takes the pressure off his spine—and keeps him from sliding off the stretcher.

Jill L. Curry, RN

Hearing aid

As a flight nurse working in a noisy environment, I've found two novel uses for my stethoscope. By placing it over a patient's trachea, I can use it to listen for air moving in and out of his chest. Also, to help hearing-impaired patients, I put the ear pieces in their ears and speak into the diaphragm.

Susan Engman, RN, MN

Diabetes supplies: Look in the book

In our hospital, some of the supplies for patients with diabetes are kept in the pharmacy and others in materials management. So I made a list of all the supplies, their order numbers, and where they're stored. We keep this list in front of the materials-management book in each unit. When someone needs a particular item, she can look on the list and then easily order it.

Julie R. Welsh, RN, MS

Comfort

Skin lotion warm-up

Here's one way to avoid applying cold skin lotion to a patient after his bath: Place the lotion bottle, with the cap tightly closed, in the patient's bathwater. As the patient warms up, so does the lotion.

This warm-water treatment also keeps the lotion from thickening.

Gail Lew, RN

Traction warm-up

A patient who's fractured his femur and is in traction may complain that his foot is cold. So I put an empty, flannel ice-bag cover over the foot to warm it up. The cover can be removed easily for circulation checks, and it won't interfere with traction.

Kim Kill, RN

Toasty toes

Toes extending from a foot cast can get awfully cold in the winter. To keep them warm and cozy, cover them with a baby's hat, tying the hat's strings around the ankle to keep the hat in place.

Marilyn McGarry, RN

Capital suggestion

To help elderly patients stay warm, encourage them to wear knit caps indoors. This will help them retain body heat and, unlike elastic socks and extra covers, won't impair circulation.

Justine C. McGill, RN

One size fits all

Many of my male patients complain about having cold heads. So I take a piece of stockinette from our cast cart and put a rubber band around the top 1" of the stockinette to close one end. Then I cuff the other end. Now I have a soft, warm cap that will stretch to fit any size head.

Isabelle L. Colomy, LPN

Warm up a cold seat

For patients who complain about sitting on a cold toilet seat, try this: Cut a large hole in a disposable underpad and lay it over the seat, absorbent side up. The patient will feel a lot more comfortable.

Teresa G. James, RN

Who wears sweatpants?

In the extended care facility where I work, most of our elderly residents get out of bed and dress every day. But the men don't wear regular trousers; they wear sweatpants with a drawstring waist. Besides being easy to put on and take off, the sweatpants are warm, comfortable, inexpensive, and easy to launder.

Joanne Breden, RN

Warming up: All arms and legs

After having surgery, I had to stay in bed for 2 weeks. Because I wore short-sleeved hospital gowns, I was occasionally chilled. So I borrowed a pair of my daughter's leg warmers and slipped them over my arms. They were perfect for warming me up and easy to remove.

Deborah Rang, LPN

Warm arms

When elderly patients complain that they're cold, I don't give them bulky sweaters; I cover their arms with leg warmers. To check vital signs or I.V. sites, I simply push the leg warmers up or down.

Terri Huncharek, LVN

Lap rap

In the nursing home where we work, some residents in wheelchairs have trouble keeping their lap robes in place. So we glued a strip of Velcro to each side of the wheel-chair and sewed corresponding Velcro strips on two edges of the lap robe. When the Velcro on the lap robe is attached to the Velcro on the wheelchair, the robe stays in place. Yet the robe can be pulled off easily if the patient must be transferred.

Sandra Magana, RN

Out of the cribs of babes

Crib blankets or coverlets are a perfect size for covering the laps and legs of people in wheelchairs. They're soft, washable, colorful— and they protect your patients' legs from cold and drafts.

Mary Hendela, RN

Durable leg warmers

Some of our women residents in wheelchairs suffer from cold legs. Their dresses don't cover their legs, and their stockings are too thin to be warm. Lap robes don't help much either; they're constantly sliding off and don't even cover the backs of the legs.

But we've found a solution to this chilling problem in leg warmers—those long footless socks that are so popular now, but were formerly worn only by dancers. Leg warmers are inexpensive, durable, and available in a variety of colors. Besides warming the lower leg, they extend well up over the knee, and stay there (yet they're not so tight that they impede circulation). And the patient doesn't have to bother taking them off when using the bathroom.

We keep several pairs of leg warmers on hand and suggest to residents' families that they make great gifts.

Nadine Hardage, CNA

Quick comfort for pregnant women

To make a woman in labor more comfortable, put a blanket in a microwave oven for 2 or 3 minutes, then apply the warm blanket to the woman's back or pubic area. The blanket holds heat well and provides quick comfort.

Beverly Jacks, RN, BSN

Warm 'n' ready

To help ensure a patient's comfort during a vaginal examination, warm up those specula.

Put a heating pad into a pillowcase, place both on the examining cart, and turn the pad to a low temperature. Then, set various-sized specula on the pillowcase and cover them with a small towel.

This guarantees your patient a bit more comfort during her examination. It also saves time because the equipment is always at the right temperature whenever you need to use it.

Catherine Lawer, RN

No more complaints

If patients complain that they dread the cold speculum during their gynecological examination, here's a way to end the complaints. Keep a jar of warm water in each examining room. Just before the doctor goes into a room, put the speculum in the water. When the doctor's ready to do the vaginal examination, he'll remove the speculum. The warm speculum helps the patient relax, and the water serves as a lubricant to make insertion easier.

Karen Starling, RN, PHN

Stirrup comfort

As any woman knows, those ob/gyn examination table stirrups can be cold, hard, and uncomfortable.

To minimize this, simply slip a pair of knitted or disposable foam slippers, bottom side up, over the stirrups.

The slippers will certainly help your patients relax. They may even prompt some patients to thank you for your thoughtfulness.

Faith Kahly, RN

Keeping a cool head

After oral surgery, most of our patients are too sleepy to hold regular ice packs on their jaws bilaterally as ordered. So we help them this way: We tie a knot in the middle of a long piece of stockinette. Then, we fill two examination gloves with ice and knot each glove at the wrist. We put the gloves in the stockinette—one on each side of the knot in the middle. Finally, we wrap the stockinette around the patient's head with the knot under his chin and the ends tied loosely on top of his head.

This stockinette ice bag stays put without being held in place. And we can easily change the ice as needed.

Sue Dillon, RN

Numb mum

A new mother who wants to breast-feed her baby but whose nipples are sore might appreciate this suggestion from you.

Just before breast-feeding, tell her to wrap some ice chips in a cloth and apply it to the nipple. In a minute or so, the nipple will be numb, the baby can start sucking, and the mother won't feel the soreness that usually accompanies the first few moments of breast-feeding. (The cold also makes the nipple more erect, so it's easier for the baby to grasp.)

Maureen A. Storey, RN

Cool comfort

For my postpartum patient, I put perineal pads in the refrigerator. When they're cool, I take one out, sprinkle it with cold water, place it next to the perineum, and then apply an ice pack. The cool pad comforts her sore perineum and protects her skin from the ice pack.

Barbara J. Whitmore, RN

Cool relief

Itchy skin under a plaster cast is a real problem for orthopedic patients. But a hand-held blow-dryer, set at the cool temperature and aimed at the problem area, readily relieves the itching.

Debbie Almes, RN

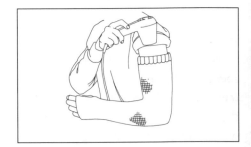

Protective clothing

A postlumpectomy patient can minimize skin discomfort and peeling by wearing a cotton camisole under her bra during the weeks she's receiving radiation treatments. This worked well for me.

Sandra Rubadeux, RN

Banding together to prevent irritation

Tape used to secure nasal "drip pads" after sinus or nasal surgery can irritate a patient's skin. So the staff on our postanesthesia care unit developed an alternative.

Loop together four or five rubber bands (depending on the size of the patient's face). Place an end over each of the patient's ears, making sure you put some padding under neath the rubber bands to prevent chafing. Then position the middle over the drip pads.

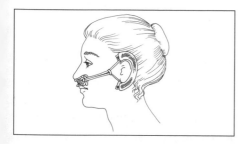

This is an inexpensive way to hold drip pads in place, and it makes dressing changes easier.
Judith Miller, RN

Curlers for comfort

Most of our coronary care unit patients receive oxygen by nasal cannula. But the part of the cannula that goes behind the ears can be uncomfortable. Here's what I did to solve the problem.

I bought foam curlers and removed the plastic part from the center of each. This left a hollow roll. I cut each curler up the side. After I put the tubing through the curler, I placed the curler behind the patient's ear. This is an inexpensive way to prevent excoriation.

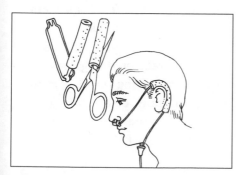

If you need to stabilize the tubing, place a small loop of tape—with the sticky side out—inside the curler.

Of course, the curlers are discarded after they're used or if they become dirty.
Sue Biley, RN

Remade masks

Many patients refuse to wear their one-size-fits-all oxygen masks because these masks are simply too large and uncomfortable: The plastic rim juts into the patient's eyes and allows air to escape.

To tailor the mask, trim the top edge a bit and cover it with cloth tape. With a comfortable custom-fit mask, the patients become more compliant with their oxygen therapy.
Jerene Maune, RN

Support system

On our respiratory intensive care unit, intubated patients used to experience discomfort from the weight of the ventilator tubing on the endotracheal tube. To correct this problem, we now put a rolled bath towel under the ventilator tubing near the endotracheal tube. This also helps keep the tube in position.
Cindy Cicerchi, RN
Cheryl McConnell, RN

Controlled relaxation

The controlled-relaxation techniques for labor and delivery taught in prepared childbirth classes can be used prenatally and postpartum, too. For example, women who have difficulty falling asleep during late pregnancy may find that controlled relaxation helps induce sleep in a short time.

Also, nursing mothers who are tense or nervous at feeding times may find that controlled relaxation works just as well as a glass of wine or beer.

Muriel A. Zraning, RN

Prep talk

In preparation for gastrointestinal diagnostic studies, a patient may need to drink castor oil or magnesium salts. To diminish the unpleasant taste of these preparations, give the patient some hard candy or gum between swallows. This sweet break also helps prevent nausea, so the patient can drink all of the liquid. If the patient is diabetic, use sugar-free candy or gum.

Wendy A. Simon, RN

Jelly warm-up

To help patients relax during sigmoidoscopies and digital examinations, warm the lubricating jelly before you apply it. Place the tube upside down in a pitcher of warm water for about 10 minutes. Then when the jelly's applied for the digital examination or sigmoidoscopy, the patient doesn't get as tense as with a cold touch.

Darlene Arnston

Rolling pin relief

Here's a practical and effective way to treat women suffering from back labor. Use two rolling pins—the hollow kind that can be filled with water. Keep one in the placenta freezer and the other at the nurse's station ready to be filled with hot water.

Place a towel on the patient's back to protect her from the extreme temperature of the rolling pin. Then, with the help of the expectant father, roll one of the pins over the woman's back. The combination of heat or cold and the gentle pressure from the rolling motion seems to give relief.

Rae K. Grad, RN

Water rings

Does your patient need an air ring? Give him a water ring instead. Just fill about three-quarters of the ring with water, expel the air, and close the cap. The water-filled ring stays soft and is more comfortable than an air ring.

In cold weather, though, you might warm up the ring in a warm-water washbowl before having the patient sit on the ring.

Pauline Seibel, RN

Water bed for the head

Concerned about the back of a patient's head when he must spend a great deal of time on his back? To relieve discomfort, fill a hot-water bottle with 2 cups of water and press out all excess air. With the water pillow under his head, the patient is more comfortable.

Myrtle L. Little, RN

Urinal comfort from a cup

When a male patient wants to keep a urinal in place, I tear off the bottom of a 6-oz foam cup and slide the tapered end into the urinal. The cup provides a soft surface for the penis, decreasing tissue trauma and increasing patient comfort. It also traps urine away from the skin, keeping the skin dry.

Barbara Dagastine, RN, EdMS

Comfortable fit for gait belt

A gait belt can be uncomfortable and may irritate a patient's skin. So I put a small towel under the belt before placing it snugly on the patient. The towel protects the skin and makes the belt more comfortable to wear.

Joy Fussy, RN

Comfort for hemorrhoid sufferers

A new mother with hemorrhoids may find that the sanitary pads she uses to absorb lochia can irritate the hemorrhoids. This is especially true when she walks. So I suggest switching to adult incontinence pads. They're more comfortable but still absorb lochia.

Maurenne E. Griese, RN, BSN

Inside out for comfort

I encourage a patient with edema to turn his antiembolism stockings inside out before putting them on. The stockings are then more comfortable because the open ridge is on the outside. That reduces pressure and friction on his foot.

Mary Solomon, RN

Open-door policy

At a nursing home that I recently visited, each resident's room had a mini-door between the real door and the hallway. The mini-door was made of fabric stretched over a wooden frame that was the width of the real door. About 2½' high, the mini-door was fastened by hinges at the side, about two-thirds of the way up the real door. This arrangement provided privacy from passersby without isolating the resident behind a closed door. Plus, the nurses could easily hear each resident from his room.

Tracie Stuart, RN

Armboard alternative

When we're preparing an intensive care unit patient for a temporary pacemaker, pulmonary artery catheter, or an antecubital I.V. line, we sometimes use a foam and nylon knee immobilizer instead of an arm-board. If necessary, we trim the fastener so we can access the insertion site.

The device can be easily secured and removed. It relieves pressure by distributing the patient's weight, and it fits comfortably when properly adjusted.

Gary Walters, RN, BSN

Taped for comfort

A dialysis patient may have sensitive skin and, if he takes minoxidil, excessive hair growth. So I try to avoid taping dialysate infusion lines to his wrists. Instead, I ask him to bring in a clean sweatband, which I place on his wrist. Then I tape the lines to the band. This will eliminate unnecessary discomfort.

Sue S. McRae, RN

Easing arthritis pain

For arthritic patients, gripping tools and utensils can be painful and difficult. I suggest that they buy foam pipe insulation and glue it to the handles. This insulation is available at hardware stores, and it comes in several diameters that can be cut to the desired length. Not only does this make gripping easier, but it also helps to reduce fatigue.

Wendy Dabney, RN

That old smoothie

You've probably heard about using a satin pillowcase to save your hairdo, but here's another idea for that old smoothie, satin.

For arthritic patients, just turning over in bed at night can be a real problem. Suggest that a satin draw-sheet be made for their beds. First, buy enough satin for the width of the bed. Then sew a strip of terry cloth or a bath towel on two ends to tuck under the mattress. Being a coarser texture, the terry cloth keeps the satin from slipping.

Roberta Steele, RN

No more numbness

When treating a patient's sore throat with an anesthetic antiseptic like Chloraseptic, you can easily get some of the spray on the patient's tongue. Then the patient's throat may feel better, but he has the discomfort of a numb tongue.

To prevent a numb tongue, invert the bowl of a teaspoon over the patient's tongue and then spray his throat. The spoon not only protects his tongue from the spray, but also depresses the tongue so you can see the area of the throat that's red and sore.

Linda Barker, RN

Soothing solution

Here's one way to relieve mouth soreness when patients undergo chemotherapy or radiotherapy. Give them yogurt. Chilled or frozen yogurt soothes the mucous membranes while providing a high-protein snack. (Both regular and diet yogurt contain 8 to 10 g of protein per 8-oz container.) Thus, yogurt also helps supply the additional energy patients need when undergoing chemotherapy or radiotherapy.

Connie Danser, RN

A hand towel

When a patient needs a hand splint, I make one that doesn't irritate his skin with a lot of tape. I just roll a small towel and tape it so it retains its rolled shape. Then I attach two Montgomery straps—one on each end of the roll. I place some gauze on the back of the patient's hand, put the rolled towel in his palm, and fasten the Montgomery straps over the gauze.

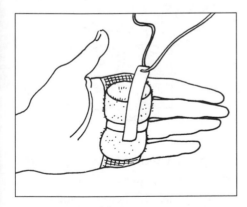

Besides being more comfortable for the patient, my hand towel splint is easier to manage than the taped-on variety.

Margie Downs, RN

Music to promote sleep

In our busy—and sometimes noisy—ICU, many patients have trouble sleeping. I have found that a cassette player with earphones, brought from home, helps drown out the noise for these patients. And when listening to their favorite music, they relax and fall asleep easier.

Capt. Marie Baudreau

Emergencies

Suction equipment: All boxed up

Because our crash cart doesn't contain all of the suction equipment we need for a code, we made up a suction box to keep on top of the cart. The box is a bright yellow toolbox that was purchased at a hardware store. We put everything needed for suctioning in the box, along with a contents list that's signed when the box is restocked. Now we don't have to search for suction equipment during an emergency.

Julie R. Welsh, RN, MS

Removing airway equipment in one step

In our hospital, we use tool chests as code carts. We place all the airway equipment in the bottom of the chest, in a plastic basin. During a code, we can quickly remove the basin and place it by the head of the patient's bed. The airway equipment is readily available, and some of the congestion around the cart is eliminated—we don't have to keep reaching into the cart to get more airway equipment.

Kate White, RN

Bee ready

Here's a way to make life easier for patients who are allergic to bee stings and must carry an anaphylaxis kit. Tell them a plastic travel toothbrush case holds the equipment compactly. Especially convenient for children, the case fits into a back pocket so it can be carried easily outdoors.

To alert others to the patient's prescribed dosage, a prescription label can be attached to the case.

Linda Dattolico, RN

Snip 'n' shrivel

When a patient has a Sengstaken-Blakemore tube in place, the esophageal balloon may slip upward, causing the patient to suffocate. As a safeguard, keep a pair of scissors taped to the head of the bed for emergencies. If immediate deflation becomes necessary, cut the inflation tube and release the pressure. Although this happens rarely, life hangs in the balance, so be prepared.

Brigid Jaynes, RN

Supportive measures

Nickel's worth

After eye surgery, a patient with dressings over both eyes may have trouble finding the nurses' call button on the bedside console. Tape a nickel on top of the button to help the patient identify it. Then he need only run his fingers over the console until he feels the familiar coin, and press the button.

Daryl Seifert, RN

For CVA patients, the cutting edge

After a cerebrovascular accident (CVA), a patient may feel frustrated by his inability to cut his food. Ask his family to bring in a pizza cutter (rolling knife). He can use it on almost any food. This may help to increase his self-esteem and independence.

Melodee Miller, RN

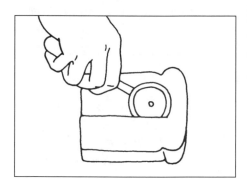

Keeping track of hearing aids

Sometimes, a patient with a hearing aid may remove it before going to the operating room. (I always check to make sure he doesn't need it to hear instructions or respond to questions.) To keep the hearing aid from getting lost, I put it inside a dental cup and cover the top. Then I write the patient's name, room number, and *hearing aid* on a piece of tape. I place the tape on the top of the cup and put the cup next to the patient's bed so that his hearing aid will be there when he returns.

Sujitra Vibulbhan, RN, BS

Only natural

When I'm preparing a patient for a craniotomy, I save a lock of his hair. If he has a hairpiece made later, he'll have a sample of his natural hair color.

Patricia Gallagher, RN, BS, MS

Simple gesture

As a nurse with alopecia, I understand the needs of other women who have this condition. When a bald woman is too ill to wear her wig, give her a scrub cap or turban to cover her head. This simple gesture will make her feel less self-conscious.

Karen W. Kasmarik, RN, BSN

Increased visibility

Many patients complain when their bed rails are padded as a seizure precaution. They say the padding prevents them from seeing out of the bed. So we now cover the rails with foam tubing used to stop dripping from sweaty water pipes. We slit the tubing lengthwise along the seam, place it on each rail, then stabilize it with duct tape. The inexpen-

sive tubing, available at any hardware store, is easy to wash and disinfect. And it doesn't get in the way when we have to raise or lower the bed rails.

Judy Sieber, RN

Aquatic therapy

In our intermediate care facility, we've found that aquariums can provide excellent visual stimulation for patients who have attention span deficits. A teenage volunteer designs and maintains the aquariums, filling them with colorful fish, plants, and rocks.

Peggy Kay-Herndon, LPN

Fill in the blanks

If you have a patient who's paralyzed or immobilized and must spend a lot of time in a side-lying position to prevent decubiti, here's a way to help him: Make an inexpensive magazine or book holder to attach to the bed so the patient can read rather than just stare at the wall. The holder is ideal for one-page articles, poems, or letters.

First, get one of those report cover kits with clear plastic sheets and plastic slide locks. (They're available at most variety stores or drugstores.) Cut two of the plastic sheets about 3" longer and 1" wider than the book or magazine that will go into the holder. Next, staple the sheets together on three sides to make an envelope or pouch.

Then, cut the slide locks to fit the envelope's sides and bottom (miter the adjoining edges of the slide locks for a tighter fit). With a hot ice pick or small drill, make two holes in each slide lock. Lace a 4-ply yarn through the holes, leaving about 8" on each side and on the bottom to loop around the top and bottom bed rails.

Finally, tie the holder to the bed rails, adjust it to the patient's eye level, and slip in the book or magazine. The holder won't hamper the bed rails' movement. Best of all, because the materials just slide in, you can vary the patient's "sideshow"—and keep boredom at bay—with just a flip of your wrist.

Pat Baggerly, RN

Notes to remember

When I'm caring for a head-trauma patient, I give him a small notebook to jot down factual information, such as the reason he's in the hospital, his doctor's name, and the time of his therapy session. I've noticed that patients who record this kind of information seem more self-confident because they don't have to repeat their questions.

Melodee Miller, RN

Circle of love

Many of our patients in the intensive care unit are on ventilators. If they're restless, they'll pick and pull at anything they can reach. We've come up with a way to keep their hands off critical tubes and wires.

Ask the patient's family members to bring in small, personal items that aren't sharp, such as a grandchild's toy. Attach them to a long piece of basting tape. Use as many items as needed, placing them about 3" apart and tying knots to separate them. Then tie the ends of the tape together to make a circle. Now the patient has something to hold— something that will remind him of his family.

Janeen F. Twohey, RN

Voice of love

I learned this valuable tip from a 13-year-old boy. It proves how important a family member's help can be in a patient's care and recovery.

One of our elderly patients, normally a good-natured man, became confused and combative after surgery. At night, he sometimes tried to climb out of bed. After we told his family about these problems, this man's 13-year-old grandson took it upon himself to make a tape recording. On the tape the boy reminded his grandfather that he was in a hospital because he needed an operation, that the surgery was over now and he'd soon be going home, and that Grandma would be there in the morning to have breakfast with him. Most important, he told his grandfather he loved him.

The boy brought the tape in and the next time his grandfather became confused, we played it for him. When he heard his grandson's familiar voice, full of tenderness and love, he calmed down and went back to sleep.

Joan Hansen, RN

Musical messages

Only family members may visit patients on our intensive care unit. That policy has been unpopular with the friends of teenage patients. To appease them, we suggest that they call the patient's favorite radio station and request that a song be played at a specific time, dedicated to their friend. We then provide a radio for the patient so he can hear his musical gift.

Patricia Bugg, RN

Weather report for ICU patients

Some patients in the intensive care unit (ICU) become confused and disoriented after being on the unit for a while. To keep them aware of the world outside, I post a sign that includes the month, day, and year, the day's temperature, and weather forecast.

Karen Fleming, LPN

Loving phone calls

I've found that phone calls to family members often cheer up my patients who are receiving chemo-therapy or radiation treatments. Here's what you can do: Post the names and phone numbers of family members in the patient's room. Then, any staff member can put the patient in touch with a friendly voice when he needs some cheering up.

Margie Schorpp, SN

Calendar of events

When a patient requires a long hospitalization, family members become discouraged. Suggest that they draw a progress calendar on a poster board and hang it in the patient's room. They can mark the calendar with stickers and encouraging comments each day, focusing on positive steps in his recovery.

Nancy Carole Munzig, RN, BSN

Perfumed room

Recently we cared for a patient who had burns on 40% of her body. Several days after admission, she began to complain about the odors coming from her burn dressings and wounds.

To alleviate this problem, the patient asked her husband to bring her favorite bottle of perfume to the hospital. He did, and each day he or a staff member sprayed the perfume into the air around her, making sure none of the perfume settled on her burn sites.

We noticed several positive effects from the perfume treatment. First, the patient wasn't bothered by the odor from her wounds any more. Second, she was buoyed by the control she exerted over her environment. And third, her husband felt a sense of participation in his wife's care.

Sue Hendricks, RN
Reginald L. Richard, PT, MS

Distraction techniques

Distracting an anxious patient can be difficult when you're giving an injection or starting an I.V. I usually try to talk with him about a subject he enjoys. If that doesn't work, I give him a simple task to concentrate on, such as wiggling his toes or alternately opening and closing his hand (the one opposite the hand or arm I'm working on). These distraction techniques will usually reduce his anxiety.

Pia H. Edgar, RN

For inquiring minds

My patients often ask about disease-related organizations and support groups. I keep this information in a pocket-sized address book, listing the organizations and groups in alphabetical order according to the disease or condition. For example, I'd find the American Cancer Society under "C" for cancer.

Judy Trainer, SN

Getting the whole picture

To understand a nursing-home patient's past, we ask his family to bring in pictures of him in various stages of life, from childhood to late adulthood. That gives us a sense of who he is—and was.

Cecilia M. Bidigare, RN,C, MSN

In-house art gallery

At the retirement home where I work, we're constantly looking for new and interesting activities for our residents. So ever since our local library began lending framed pictures to its cardholders, we've been borrowing two pictures a month and hanging them in the hall. The residents enjoy studying the art and following up their study with a lively discussion. They look forward to our new acquisitions each month.

Marilyn Moore, RN

Polished plan

Ever try conducting a manicure session for elderly patients? You'll be surprised how a simple activity like this can generate fun and interest.

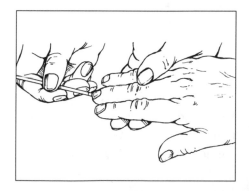

As an added benefit, manicuring offers an opportunity to encourage finger movement.

Evelyn R. White, RN

Transferring patients: The right directions

I work in the emergency department of a rural hospital. Occasionally, we have to transfer a patient to one of seven larger facilities in the area. All are at least 45 minutes away, so we keep directions to them available for our patients' families. Knowing exactly where to go helps ease their anxiety during the trip.

Lori F. Hall, RN, CEN, BSN

Help for grieving adults

"People ask me how my mom's doing since dad died—but not how I'm doing. And I lost my father!"

That comment, and others like it, inspired a nurse and a social worker to form support groups for adults who've had a parent die recently. A clinical nurse specialist and thanatologist at St. Luke's Hospital, Milwaukee, and a social worker at Lutheran Social Services, Milwaukee, hold these group meetings to help adults understand, accept, and deal with the death of a parent.

The groups, each with about 10 participants, meet once a week for 6 consecutive weeks. At the 1 ½- to 2-hour sessions, participants talk about their feelings, their relationship with the surviving parent, and topics of special interest to them, such as sibling disagreements or a child's grief. They also watch and discuss a filmstrip on death and mourning, and receive handouts that explain stress, grief, and guilt.

Among the techniques used is one in which participants list five things they enjoy doing and five things they find stressful, then decide how often they did these things within the last month, week, and 24 hours. This exercise makes the grievers aware of what makes them feel good and helps them avoid what depresses them. Participants also learn breathing exercises, deep muscle relaxation, and other techniques they can use when they feel stressed.

At the final meeting, participants share wine and cheese and receive "gifts"—positive statements about themselves from the other group members. Many also exchange addresses and phone numbers for future contacts. Before they leave, the participants evaluate the sessions. Their responses have included: "The group helped bring me out of a prolonged state of shock and denial," "I feel I can cope now," and "I've learned that I'm not alone."

Virginia Bourne, RN, MSN
Judy Meier, MSW

4 PEDIATRIC PATIENT CARE

Fluid and nutrition

Technique to help a baby breast-feed

A new mother on our obstetric unit was having trouble breast-feeding her baby because her nipples weren't large enough to induce the sucking response.

So we cut a regular disposable nipple in half lengthwise and placed part of it on top of the mother's nipple. The nipple provided enough stimulation to help the baby suck. The mother held onto the nipple until her baby began nursing, then she gently pulled it away.

This technique allowed her to breast-feed her baby and ended her frustration.

Dawn Denton, RN

A picture worth an ounce of fluid

In our pediatric unit, we give a postoperative patient a 1-oz medicine cup and a coloring sheet with 10 pictures on it. Each time a child finishes drinking 1 cup of fluid, he may color an item on the sheet. When he's colored all the pictures, we discontinue his I.V. line.

This encourages the child to drink fluid and lets him have fun, too.

Connie Rawls, RN

Lemon sips and chips

On the pediatric unit where I work, we had a young boy who underwent an appendectomy. He didn't want to drink water with ice chips (as ordered), but he liked the taste of lemon glycerin swabs. So I squeezed the juice from a few swabs into his ice water. He enjoyed the "treat" while also complying with his doctor's order.

Michael Dimsey, Corpsman, U.S. Navy

Contest for kids

I encourage a child to drink after a tonsillectomy or adenoidectomy by pouring his liquid in a plastic medication cup. This cup is less intimidating than a larger drinking cup, so he's more likely to drink from it. Then I have a contest to see how many cups he can drink each hour.

Debbie Thomas, RN

Keeping score

To encourage pediatric patients to take fluids after surgery, devise an attractive "scorecard."

Draw on a sheet of paper various symbols representing fluids: soda bottles, flavored ice pops, ice cream, flavored gelatin, milk, and water. After the child takes the fluid, he colors the appropriate symbol on his scorecard.

Martha Clark, RN

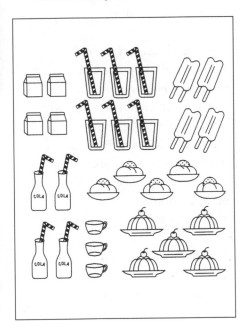

Down the spout

Getting bedridden patients to drink used to cause more fluid spilled than consumed, especially with tots who haven't quite mastered drinking through straws, or with postoperative patients who aren't allowed straws. Eliminate the mess by using special drinking cups—the kind that with sipper lids. They can be found in most grocery stores or drugstores. So, if a patient can raise his head, he can drink—unassisted and unafraid of spilling.

Diane Voellner, RN, MN

Circuitous solution

Getting small children to force fluids can be a problem. Use plastic "crazy straws," which are constructed in complicated shapes. The youngsters love watching the path of the juice when they sip. They take adequate fluids and won't let the straw out of sight.

Dianne Charron, RN

Perfect timing

Getting a child to void or drink at a certain time usually requires a little ingenuity. As an incentive, we use a kitchen timer.

For example, if a child must give a second-voided specimen in 20 minutes, or drink fluids every hour, we set the timer accordingly. While it's ticking away, the child mentally prepares himself for the task at hand. When the timer goes off, the child knows that he's "on," and usually performs with great enthusiasm.

Candy Pollack, RN

Play therapy

Put up a happy face

To increase visual stimulation for infants who require restraint (such as those undergoing cleft lip repair), tape pictures of happy, smiling faces inside their cribs. Toothpaste advertisements in magazines are especially good, and the little ones seem to enjoy gazing at human faces.

Rita A. Fleming, RN

Bouncy mobile

Here's a way to make a colorful, inexpensive mobile to stimulate infants and bedridden youngsters. Punch eight holes in a paper or foam dinner plate, making a circular pattern. Cut a long piece of string into four 24" pieces; then thread each piece up through the bottom of the plate and down through the next hole.

Now you can be creative. Cut animal pictures from magazines, or make snowflakes or other shapes from colored paper, and tie your creations to the strings hanging from the plate. To suspend the mobile, just punch two more holes in the center of the plate, and thread a strong rubber band through the holes, tying it to a long string at the top. Then tape the string to the ceiling or hang it from the I.V. pole.

The rubber band makes the animals and snowflakes dance if the child pulls on the mobile, and gives the plate some bounce so it won't tear easily.

Sylvia Spearr, RN

Exit ennui

Boredom and short attention spans are problems in pediatrics.

Use a "Game Crash Cart" filled with cards, crayons, books, tracing paper, puppets, and other toys liked by both boys and girls of all ages. The gaily decorated cart creates an air of excitement and joy for bedridden patients. It's an orderly way of keeping many diversionary objects available for the children.

Joanne Serapilia, SN

Cookie cutters for kids

Blunt-edged plastic cookie cutters make safe, inexpensive toys for pediatric patients. They also work great for cutting shapes from toast, gelatin, or blocks of ice cream (for those children who need encouragement to eat). You can easily disinfect the cookie cutters—and some brands can even withstand autoclaving.

Terrilynn Quillen, RN

Child's play: Double dressings

A favorite stuffed animal or doll can comfort a pediatric patient. When

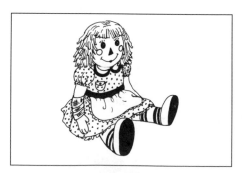

the child has surgery, we put a similar dressing on his stuffed animal. The patient feels less lonely, and we can initiate play therapy more easily.

Joan O'Connor, RN

Everybody wins

If you do skin tests on children, make the testing less traumatic by using this guessing game.

First, divide the child's back into sections according to the different types of allergens (weeds, trees, and so on). Next, ask both the child and his parent to guess how many allergy extract drops you'll administer in each section.

Then, as you administer the drops, count them. If someone guesses the exact number, he gets two points. If neither parent nor child guesses correctly, the player with the closest guess gets one point. The player with the highest score wins. Repeat the game for each section of the child's back, until the allergy testing is complete.

The game lets the child relax between administrations and diverts his attention from the test. The few minutes you spend explaining the game beforehand save many minutes of fighting, crying, and struggling. So, really, everyone—child, parent, and nurse—wins.

Beverly Opitz, RN

Body painting

If you have a hard time putting calamine lotion on wiggling, squirming children, try my method. Get a small paintbrush and paint the child's skin with the lotion. Most children love the novelty of having their body painted, and they'll be sure to sit still during the procedure.

Kathy Dougherty, RN

Soaking procedure

In the busy emergency department where I work, I frequently have to soak a child's finger or hand wound. But just as frequently, I run out of basins for the soaking solution.

Then I use a clean plastic urine container instead. The container is transparent, so I play finger games with the child to encourage him to move his fingers or hand for a more thorough cleansing.

Mary Eggen, RN

Mobility

Color-coded crutches for children

When a child is learning how to use crutches, I tie yarn bows to his shoes and crutches. I use one color for the right shoe and crutch and another color for the left shoe and crutch (as shown on the next page). This will make the experience easier and more fun.

Rita K. Spillane, RN

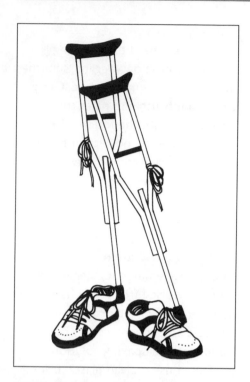

Help for handicapped tots

To help a handicapped toddler learn to walk, make a set of sturdy, economical parallel bars from wooden dowels and ordinary kitchen chairs.

At a lumber company, buy two 8' dowels, 1" in diameter. Sand and varnish the dowels and attach a piece of clothesline to each end with a small nail. Then place the dowels over the seats of two kitchen chairs and tie the ends of the dowels to the chair backs. The height and width of the chair seats are just right for a toddler.

When the bars aren't in use, untie them and put them away.
Helen Hoke, RN

Children only, please

Do you use oversized wheelchairs or large carts to transport children from the pediatrics unit to other areas of the hospital? This often adds to their fright in unfamiliar surroundings.

To make this experience as pleasant as possible, use a large red wagon that comfortably carries children up to the age of about 9. Since most children have a wagon at home, it gives them something to relate to and makes their trip a happier experience.
Barbara Berger, RN
Barbara Jurgelis, RN

Skin care

It's oil for the better

To remove the vernix caseosa from a newborn's skin, use mineral oil. Just soak some gauze or a cotton ball with the oil and wipe clean.
Irma Robinson, LPN

Tops on bottoms

I was recently given a challenging order in the special-care nursery: to expose to room air the red, sore buttocks of a 4½-lb premature infant without risking temperature loss. Since she was in an open crib, I was afraid that if I left her uncovered from the waist down, she'd get too cold. So instead, I put another undershirt on her—a bit differently, though. I put the baby's legs through the arms of this undershirt and left her buttocks exposed through the neck opening.

The baby's mother was amused when she visited and found undershirts on *both* ends of her little girl. But she was glad to learn that her baby was warm while her buttocks were healing.

Ellyn Presley, LPN, EMT

Smooth change for newborns

To prevent meconium from sticking to a newborn's sensitive skin, spread petroleum jelly on his clean bottom. This will protect his skin and make his diaper change easier.

Susan E. Droulette, RN

Handy way to treat diaper rash

In the newborn nursery where I work, we treat diaper rash with plain water and a soft cloth. We recommend that mothers use the same method at home, using inexpensive cloth wipes as the soft cloth. We tell them to wash and dry the wipes first. Then, after using the wipes, they can wash them again or just throw them away.

Rebecca Williamson, RN

Protecting preemies' skin after surgery

A premature baby who's had intra-abdominal surgery may need frequent dressing changes. Because the tape used to secure the dressing could excoriate the baby's fragile skin, we've come up with an alternative.

We lay the baby on an open surgical mask, then loosely cross and tie the straps of the mask over the dressing. To change the dressing, we

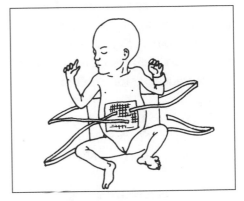

gently untie the straps. We have easy access to the wound without harming the skin.

Kay J. Bandell, RN

Knee protection for preemies

A premature baby spends a lot of time in the prone position, so delicate skin on his knees can easily tear or become abraded. I've found that disposable electrodes provide great protection because they have a jellied cushion that doesn't irritate the skin. I remove the wires and stick the electrodes to the baby's knees. The electrodes can be removed easily, and they can also be reapplied if they come off.

Eileen Cappels, RN,C

Preventing traction reaction

An orthopedic surgeon gave me a tip for preventing blisters on the heels and ankles of pediatric patients in Buck's or Bryant's traction. First, paint the affected leg with tincture of benzoin to toughen the skin. Then wrap the leg with web roll, followed by foam strips. Finally, wrap the leg in an elastic bandage.

Now you're ready to add the appropriate weights. Don't forget to check frequently for skin breakdown.

Always get a doctor's order before using this procedure.

Margaret P. Carson, RN, MS

Allergen alternative

Here's what I did when a 3-year-old patient needed a gastrostomy tube—but was allergic to tape.

I cut a piece of stockinette and slid it over his head to his abdomen to hold the dressing in place. The stockinette also held the tube close to the child's body and kept him from pulling on it.

Kim Kindred, RN

Physical care

No more tangled tubing

Our fetal heart monitor leads were constantly tangled. So I sewed two pieces of Velcro 4" long to strips of material. Then I placed each lead in the middle of the material and folded the Velcro together so that the ends attached to each other. The material is washed after each use.

Now the lines are easy to keep separate, saving both time and patience.

Linda Pfaefflin, RN, CNM

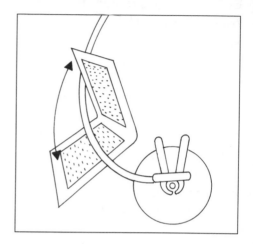

Baby boon

Sometimes administering medication to an infant can be very difficult—even with the aid of special spoons and syringes. Here's an easier way.

Put the medication in the baby's bottle and add water to make 1 oz. (Check first to see if the medication can be diluted in water.) Use a regular nipple for clear medications such as cough medicines and acetaminophen drops; use a crosscut nipple with larger holes for unclear medications that are more viscous. You can add more water to any medication left in the bottle, and make sure the baby drinks it all. Don't mix medication with formula, milk, or juice because of the risk of a drug incompatibility.

Marcy Portnoff Gever, RPh, MEd

Bright socks for baby

When suctioning an infant at home, put brightly colored socks on his hands. This will distract him, so you won't have active hands in your way. If you have to suction an infant in the hospital, ask his parents to bring in a bright pair of socks from home.

Cathy L. Wilt, LPN

Syringe alternative to suction catheters

On our neonatal unit, we use standard #6 and #8 French suction catheters to suction endotracheal tubes, but they aren't always effective. So we take a tuberculin syringe, remove the plunger and needle, and cut off the wings at the plunger end. Now the syringe fits into the suction tubing and makes it easier to suction thick oral secretions.

This works better than using a larger catheter. Remember to change the syringe as frequently as you would any other oral suctioning device.

Patrice Herberholz, RN

Mucus trap for measurement

Many of our critically ill infants have nasogastric (NG) tubes. Because they're at risk for dehydration, they may need secretion replacement. But obtaining accurate secretion measurements from large suction containers can be difficult.

I've solved this problem by placing a mucus trap in the system. Attach one end of the trap onto the NG tube and the other end onto the intermittent suction tube. (You may need an adapter, depending on the equipment you use.) This will help you with accurate fluid measurement.

Nancy Mueller, RN, BSN

Measuring drainage

To measure nasogastric drainage from newborns and small children quickly and accurately, place a mucus trap between the suction and the nasogastric tubing. You don't have to open the closed drainage system. Just check the amount and tip the trap to empty it into the suction bottle. This will be especially helpful when you can't easily estimate a small volume.

Wendy Dabney, RN

Infant allergy alert

I regularly cared for a baby with severe allergies. Because safety-alert necklaces can be dangerous for babies, I came up with a different way of alerting the staff.

I used red fabric paint to write "Severe allergies—check with nursing first" on a small bib that the baby wore. The bib warned staff members as well as volunteers of the baby's condition—they couldn't miss it—so I felt more at ease.

Susan Stewart, LPN

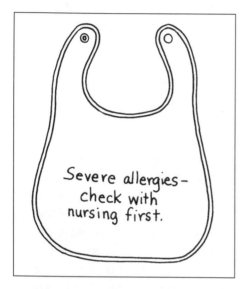

Specimen regimen

I work in a pediatrician's office where we do some of our own laboratory work, including urinalysis. We've found that urine collection bags don't work well on infants. Either they don't stay in place, or, if they're not secured properly on the infant's body, stool contaminates the specimen.

So we've devised another way to collect a sterile urine specimen. One person holds the child under both arms perpendicular to the examination table. Another person cleans the child's genital area with

sterile wipes and holds a sterile urine container under the child. The wiping stimulates urination and within a minute or so, we have our specimen.

This method of getting a clean-catch urine specimen has become standard practice for our office now.

Pat Soukup, RN

Miniature urinal

How many times have you used a urine collection bag on a premature male infant, only to have the bag slip off the infant's penis?

Here's a more effective urine collector: a capped syringe, with the needle and plunger removed. After inserting the infant's penis through the syringe's open end, place a strip of hypoallergenic tape over the closed end. Then, tape the syringe to the infant's lower abdomen or groin.

With this miniature urinal, you don't lose any of the infant's urine sample. So you get enough urine for testing, and you can measure intake and output accurately. Also, you can see the penis through the clear, plastic syringe, to check for pressure.

Nancy J. Urich, RN, BS

A collector's item

Need to get a urine specimen from an infant or toddler? Apply a pediatric urine collection bag. But if you put a diaper over the bag, you risk squeezing the bag and causing the baby discomfort as well as having urine leak out. A safer, more comfortable alternative is this:

Make a large X-shaped slash in the diaper at the front of the crotch, place the collection bag and diaper on the baby, and gently pull the bag out through the X-shaped opening. This way, there's no pressure on the bag, and you can readily see when the baby has voided.

Rose Marie Utley, RN, CPNP

Collecting urine with a condom catheter

In my unit, we designed a urine collection system for male infants and small boys that works really well. Here's what we do:

First, we place a small condom catheter over the infant's penis.

Then, we cut a hole in the center of a large transparent dressing and place the dressing over the penis so that the edges of the condom are secured at the base of the penis. We reinforce the dressing with several strips of transparent dressing (cut lengthwise) by wrapping the strips around the base of the condom to create a seal.

Finally, we connect a urine drainage system to the condom catheter and tape it securely. This system lasts for 12 hours without leaking, but comes off easily after it's soaked in water. Plus, it eliminates the need to sedate the patient or use an invasive procedure.

Jacqueline Jeffries, RN, BSN

Soaking up a urine specimen

When I have to obtain a urine specimen for a dipstick test from a young child who wears diapers, I put a cotton ball on the patient's urinary meatus or penis. I cover the cotton ball with a carefully padded plastic cover that nipples are packaged in. Then I replace the diaper. When the patient voids, the cotton ball becomes saturated with urine. This saves us from using a bag collection device each time we want to test glucose or protein levels.

Kathleen Thompson, RN

Diaper dilemma

In the pediatrician's office where I work, we frequently need to obtain stool samples for culturing from very young children with chronic diarrhea. If the child is wearing a disposable diaper, it's difficult to obtain the sample because the diaper absorbs everything. So we ask the mothers to line the diapers with plastic wrap before bringing their children in.

Laurie Quist, LPN

Quick change for blue pads

Blue pads, or disposable underpads, make a great surface for changing a baby's diaper. When a new mother goes home, tell her to take her unused pads along and keep them in her diaper bag. They'll come in handy when she needs to change her baby in a rest room or at a friend's home.

Debra J. Harries, SN

Hat trick

To keep a newborn's head warm and prevent heat loss, make him a cap from an 8" piece of stockinette. Put a rubber band around one end of the stocking to close it, roll up the other end 1" to make a cuff, and place the cap on the baby. You can also use the cap to keep a baby's head dry when he's in an oxygen hood.

Mary Kraft, RN, BSN

Baby warm-ups

To regulate a newborn's body temperature, I use two long-sleeved infant T-shirts—one to keep his arms and chest warm and the other to keep his legs and torso warm. I find that the infant becomes warmer in no time.

Linda L. Dinges, RN

Heeling warmth

Before sticking a newborn's heel for blood work, try this:

Wet the absorbent side of a dis-posable diaper with warm water. Fold the diaper in half—with the wet part inside—and place the plastic side against the newborn's heel and calf. Use the tabs to hold the diaper in place. The plastic will stay warm for at least 5 minutes without wetting or burning the skin. The newborn's heel and calf will be warmed, promoting good vasodilation.

Rena Tolbert, RN

Fancy footwork

Have you ever had to do repeated heel sticks on a crying infant to get enough blood for a specimen? If so, hold the baby's feet in warm water for 5 to 10 minutes. (Better still, let the baby's parent do the soak.) Then, with just one stick, you should be able to draw an adequate specimen.

Johnnie Titus, RN, BSN

Finger soaks are child's play

My 2-year-old son resisted warm finger soaks for cellulitis—until I added plastic toys to the water. Then he played happily while complying with the doctor's order.

Carolyn Kross, RN

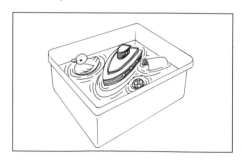

Water play for hand burns

Here's a first-aid suggestion for relieving minor hand burns in young patients.

Keep some colored, plastic ice cube containers, preferably the kind shaped like letters or numbers, in the freezer. When a child burns his hand, place the cubes in a bowl of cool water and tell the child to "catch" the shapes.

Linda S. Fish, RN, BSN

Superspenders

We recently cared for a 6-month-old baby who suffered burns on his torso. We applied dressings, then wrapped an elastic bandage over the dressings. The baby was so active, though, that the bandage kept sliding down his torso.

To keep the dressings and bandage in place, we applied two Montgomery straps to the bandage

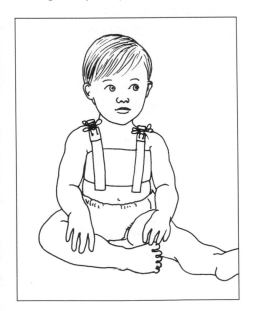

on the child's chest and the two corresponding Montgomery straps to the bandage on the child's back. Then we tied each strap—suspender style—at the baby's shoulder.

The Montgomery straps held the dressings securely in place, didn't irritate the baby's skin, and could be covered by clothing.

Frances Wartella, RN, CEN

Cap it off

When children have a sutured laceration on the scalp with a dressing that needs to be kept clean, use a bathing cap. Choose one that's a size large than needed, and it will keep the bandage clean and secure. The caps come in decorative colors so children can pretend they're airplane pilots with their rubberized headgear.

Ann Cunningham, RN

Stretch bandages for babies

I've found two ways to use net-like stretch bandages in our nursery.

One baby who needed phototherapy cried and fussed unless she was being held. So I made a "body sock" out of the stretch bandage. I placed her inside the sock, then tucked her arms in close to her body. The bandage didn't obstruct the light, and she lay quietly in her incubator.

Another baby had a fractured clavicle. To stabilize the bone, I pinned the shirtsleeve of his affected arm to the front of his shirt. But he was so strong that he could lift up his shirt. So I came up with this alternative: I secured his shoulder and arm to his body with a piece of the bandage. This worked well—his arm stayed immobile until his clavicle healed.

Shirley Worth, LPN

Straps: Banded together

Next time you have to apply Montgomery straps to a patient's incision area, don't bother with safety pins or twill tape. Instead, reach for some rubber bands and paper clips.

Slip one end of a rubber band through one of the strap's holes, then through the other end of the rubber band to secure it to the strap. Slip another rubber band through the opposite hole and secure it the same way. Then join the two rubber bands with a paper clip. Do the same with the rest of the holes in the strap.

The rubber bands allow the strap to expand as the patient moves. And since the paper clips lie flat, they won't dig into the patient's skin as a safety pin might if it popped open.

Barbara E. A. Naunchek, RN

Cast offs

"When is my cast coming off?" is a question pediatric patients ask repeatedly. But since many patients have only a vague concept of time, invent a visual aid to help them count the days: calendar cards.

Number a set of cards—one card for each day the child has to wear his cast—and hang them above his bed, like a mobile. The patient can remove one card each day, and see the numbers get smaller, or can count the remaining cards to see how many days are left. As the number of cards decreases, the number of smiles increases!

Linda Wyszinski, RN

Flower power

Have you ever had to assess the lung sounds of 2- and 3-year-old patients? Often they don't understand what to do when you tell them to take a deep breath. Or they may be too frightened to cooperate.

To get them to breathe deeply, give them a brightly colored plastic flower and ask them to smell it. Since they're familiar with flowers, they're not frightened. In fact, most children will smell it several times if necessary.

Besides eliminating the child's fears, you'll make the examination easier for yourself, too.

Joan Turner, RN, BSN

Inventive incentives

Need some incentive to get your pediatric patients to use incentive spirometers? Try this: Make a loop out of one end of a pipe cleaner. Dip the loop into some diluted baby shampoo. Then ask the child to take a deep breath and blow into the loop. He'll love the bubbles—and you'll love his sudden compliance with breathing exercises.

Cindy Sanders, RN

Here's another variation of the same idea. Attach a surgical glove to the top of a 60-ml syringe. Have the patient put the tip of the syringe in his mouth. Then encourage him to blow up the glove. He'll enjoy counting each finger as it blows up with air. (Of course, you should closely monitor the child when he practices this or any other breathing exercise.)

Patricia McShane, RN

This idea may also work. Wrap some thin paper (such as onionskin typing paper or tissue paper) around a comb. Give the comb to the child and ask him to "make music" by blowing on it.

Jennie Brown, LPN

Tubing toy

Children will be more inclined to do deep-breathing exercises if you try to make them fun. A piece of disposable corrugated plastic tubing, such as those found on ventilator hookups and intermittent positive pressure breathing machines, can be used as both a toy and a spirometer.

Let the child pretend the tubing is a telescope, a whirling musical instrument, or a giant straw. If the tubing captures his imagination as a toy, he'll be more likely to cooperate in using it as a spirometer.

Terrilynn M. Quillen, RN

Pinwheel power

Here's a way to get a child to breathe deeply so you can auscultate his lungs. Give him a colorful pinwheel to play with. You can auscultate his lungs as he takes deep breaths to make the wheel spin.

Christine M. McGrath, RN

Keep it elevated

In our postanesthesia care unit, we keep a child's limb elevated by taping it to the elevating material, such as pillows or blankets. The child can maintain some independence and still keep the limb elevated to assist circulation and pain control.

Debrah Ray, RN

Stay-put ice packs

When a baby gets an injection in his thigh muscles, here's how to prevent swelling. Cover a small ice bag with a cloth and slip it into the leg of his footed pajamas. No further securing is necessary; the pajamas are snug enough to hold the ice bag in place.

Linda Barker, RN

Offering an icy alternative

If a child won't let you apply ice to his swollen lip, offer him a flavored ice pop instead. He'll probably be more receptive to the treat than to the ice.

Myra Horn, RN

Apnea monitoring: Heart and sound

Many patients on our pediatric floor need apnea monitoring. Before, we didn't have a way to quickly locate the patient whose alarm was sounding. Here's what we did.

We bought wooden hearts at a craft store, glued magnets to the back of them, and painted them red.

Then we drew an electrocardiogram strip on each. We place them on the doors of the appropriate rooms. Now when we hear an alarm, we just look for the doors with the red hearts.

Janet Green, RN, BSN

Gloves and tape don't mix

On the neonatal intensive care unit where I work, we frequently restart I.V.s and must wear gloves. Because the tape we use to secure the I.V. sticks to the gloves, attaching the I.V. to the patient is difficult, if not impossible.

Here's our solution: Before putting on gloves, we cut a longer-than-usual piece of tape. Then we turn down each end of the tape to make a nonsticky tab. This gives us something to grab without getting our gloves stuck to the tape. With gloves on, we can then tape the I.V. in place as usual and snip off the tabs.

This tip comes in handy whenever you have to work with adhesives while wearing gloves.

Robin K. Montvilo, RN, PhD

Ease for I.V.s

I find that starting an I.V. on a squirming infant may be tricky, so I tape his arm or leg to an arm board first. Securing the catheter after cannulation is easier if the arm is already immobilized.

Kathryn E. Ausprung, RN, BSN

Keeping a child's I.V. intact

A pediatric patient with an I.V. in the antecubital fossa may have difficulty remembering not to bend his elbow. I've found that this tip works well:

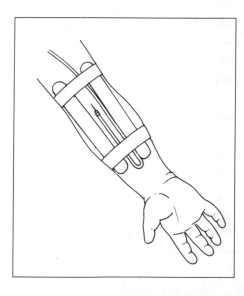

Place a tongue blade vertically on each side of the site. Then place a piece of tape horizontally across the top and bottom of both tongue blades. You'll still be able to check his I.V., but he won't be able to bend his arm.

Patty Swetnam, RN

Saline fill for a newborn's I.V.

In most cases, we use a 26-gauge angiocath if a newborn needs I.V. therapy. But when using a "dry" needle—a needle that hasn't been filled with solution—there may not be any blood return. I've found that filling the I.V. angiocath set with sterile saline solution before inserting the needle will provide a flashback of blood when the needle enters the vein. This makes it easier to start an I.V. on a newborn.

Bonnie White, RN, BSN

Airway innovations

I use plastic oral airways to help stabilize arterial lines in pediatric patients. First, I cut the flange off the convex side, then cover the airway with a 4" x 4" gauze pad. I then select the airway size that will sufficiently immobilize the patient's wrist and maintain proper flexion without causing discomfort.

Katherine McKenna, RN, CCRN

Big foot

Here's what I did to encourage pediatric patients to willingly step up on a scale to be weighed. Using a stencil and spray paint, I painted two large red footprints on the base of the scale. I even added black enamel toenails. The children usually cooperate now when I ask them to "put their feet on the big red feet."

Emilie Bonnie Daigre, RN

No more pressure

As a nurse who works in a pediatrician's office, I find that most preschoolers become anxious when they hear the words "blood pressure." So when I take a child's blood pressure, I simply show her the cuff (colorfully decorated) and say, "I need to give your arm a gentle hug with this arm band." I explain that I'll "listen" to her arm with my stethoscope. As I inflate the cuff, I say, "There's that hug."

Because the child relaxes, I get a more accurate reading. Many children ask, "Can we do it again?"

Wendy Kaveney, RN, BSN

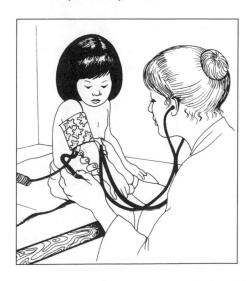

Giving injections: Tight hold

I've found a good way to give a child an intramuscular injection: Have him sit on the edge of the bed, his legs slightly apart. Ask one of his parents to stand between the child's legs and hug him. The parent should keep his or her arms over the child's arms. When you give the injection, the child can't see the needle. He's securely restrained, and he has the extra comfort of holding onto Mom or Dad.

Sandy Ringwall, RN

Distraction tactic

Here's how I take the "sting" out of pediatric injections. Before I give the injection, I hand the child an adhesive bandage and ask him to cover the exact spot where the needle goes in, right after I give the shot. The child is amazed at how hard it is to find the injection site, and this distraction helps keep him calm.

Melissa Lebon, SN

ED Story time

I keep various children's books in our emergency department (ED) so parents can use them to distract their children. For example, if a child's receiving sultures, I encourage his parents to read to him. Usually, the child becomes so interested in the story that he forgets about the procedure.

Joyce Rambo, LPN

Length wise

To measure the length of a squirming baby when you don't have a measuring board or someone to help hold the measuring tape or baby, use examination table paper. Lay the baby on the paper, hold him still with one hand, and mark the paper at the top of his head and at his heel. Be sure his leg is extended. Then remove the baby and measure the length between the two marks.

Janette Hoffman, RN, BSN

Floating faces

Ever give a baby a tepid sponge bath to reduce a high fever? Then you know what a fuss they can put up when you place them in the tub.

Next time, take some medicine cups and draw funny faces on them with an indelible marker. Then let the cups float in the water. The baby will quickly become distracted by the cups and will enjoy playing with them during the bath.

Margaret P. Carson, RN, MS

Hair-washing help

Washing the hair of a 6-year-old girl who had a myelomeningocele with an external ventricular shunt was a challenge. How could I keep the shunt collection bag even with her head?

After padding an overbed table with bedspreads, I raised it to sink level. I placed the patient on the table in a supine position and rolled her to the sink. Another nurse carried the shunt bag and I.V. My colleague stood on one side and I stood on the other and washed the girl's hair. This saved us from dragging around supplies, from soaking the bed, and from straining our backs. And our patient loved the chance to be out of bed.

Clarice Jones Tate, RN

In a doll's eye

Children hate eyedrops—and who can blame them? When my daughter needed drops for an eye infection, I got her to cooperate by first letting her put a drop in her favorite doll's eye. She saw that the doll didn't seem to mind, so she let me put a drop in her eye.

Carol Wilcox, RN

Earigation

Next time you irrigate a child's ear, try this. Use a 20-ml syringe with an I.V. plastic cannula (such as Cathalon 4) instead of the traditional irrigating syringe. This smaller syringe is softer, more pliable, and less frightening to your patient.

W.A.C. MacDonald, MB, ChB

Comfort

Warm wrap

To reduce the risk of hypothermia in an infant scheduled for surgery, I take Webril (the soft inner lining used in casting) and wrap it around his extremities. Then I put a small piece of tubular stockinette on his head in place of a surgical cap. This keeps the infant comfortable and warm.

Kay Bandell, RN

Body cast dilemma: Staying clean

When my 2-year-old son was in a body cast for 2 months, I kept the perineal area of his cast clean and dry with disposable diapers for newborns. I tucked the diaper tightly into the cast's perineal opening to prevent wetness from soaking into the cast. After 2 months, the cast had no odor or stains.

Sheryl Knoedler, RN, BSN

Diaper's on, pressure's off

Here's a technique we've devised for toddlers who've had hypospadias surgery. Although they usually have a suprapubic or perineal catheter, they still need to wear a diaper for bowel movements. But to protect the penile operative site or dressing from pressure by the diaper, we make the following modification.

We cut an X shape in the front half of a regular disposable diaper. Then we cut the bottom from a Styrofoam cup and insert the cup through the X until the rim is flush with the inside of the diaper. We tape the cup in place on the outside of the diaper.

Now the diaper can be fastened securely around the baby's waist without putting pressure on the penile dressing. And we can easily check the dressing by looking through the bottom of the cup.

Lois S. Chin, RN

Postop pointers
A pediatric patient who came to our unit after eye surgery had post-operative orders for ice packs on both eyes, 30 minutes on and 30 minutes off, for 6 hours. When we tried to comply with the orders, the patient balked at the discomfort. Then we discovered a suitable alternative.

We soaked several cotton balls in water, froze them, and substituted them for the ice packs. We had to change them frequently, but the patient didn't mind because they were softer, smaller, and not as heavy as regular ice packs.

Nancy McStay, RN

Take a breather, kid
My 5-year-old niece has unlimited confidence in my nursing abilities. When she recently suffered from an intestinal virus with frequent attacks of vomiting, my reputation was put to the test. Though I couldn't prevent the vomiting, I decided to put my knowledge of relaxation techniques to work. I taught her basic breathing exercises and imagery techniques (how to imagine relax-ing, calm scenes). With her energy and attention diverted from "being sick," she felt better and more in control of the situation.

I learned how successful my teaching had been when she later suffered a minor injury and automatically started the breathing exercises on her own. And when she was sad because her grandmother was leaving, she said, "Tell me something happy to think about so I'll feel better. I already tried puppy dogs, rainbows, and flowers, but they're not working."

Pediatric nurses can try this when their patients undergo painful procedures.

Sr. Carol Taylor, RN, MSN

Emergencies

Color-coding for pediatric emergencies
We use color-coded cards and plastic bags to prepare for pediatric emergencies in advance. The cards include emergency drug dosages, concentrations, flow rates, and defibrillator energy settings for each weight range. When a patient is admitted, we select the colored card that coincides with his weight and place it at the head of his bed. For example, if he weighs 3 to 7.25 kg (6.6 to 16 pounds), his card would be yellow. And emergency drugs and appropriately sized equipment for a patient weighing 3 to

7.25 kg are kept in a yellow plastic bag on the crash cart. This saves our staff from searching for drugs and equipment during emergencies.

Margery Lebel, RN, CCRN

Bright sights

Each patient room in our pediatric division has a large, brightly painted wooden animal propped against the wall. The puppies, frogs, bears, and other creatures delight our patients. But—more important—they make an easily accessible board to place beneath a child during a code.

Karen Pasley, RN

Milk *is* a natural

As you know, children are forever getting their teeth knocked out. But did you know that immediately replanting a tooth is the best way to preserve the tooth's life?

One course of action is to replace the tooth in its socket and ask the child to hold it in place until you get him to his dentist's office or the hospital emergency department.

Another is to try a cold glass of milk—not to drink, though. Instead, place the tooth in the cold milk. Then get the child (and the glass of milk and tooth) to the emergency department or dentist's office as quickly as possible.

Milk's osmolality keeps the root cells from enlarging or shrinking. By immersing the tooth in milk, more than half its cells will be kept alive,

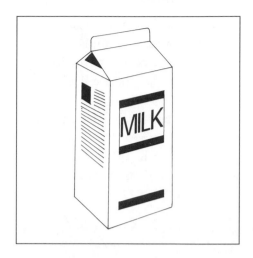

even after 12 hours. If the tooth is left out in the air (on a table, for instance), most of its cells will die within 18 minutes.

So for healthy teeth, milk really *is* a natural.

Ronald Johnson, DDS

Rx for emergencies

Standard equipment on our ambulance includes a box of lollipops. Young children seem to accept our help more readily if we greet them with a lollipop in hand, rather than with unfamiliar, scary-looking emergency equipment.

Ann Hauser, BA, EMT-P

Cart smarts

We keep a small three-shelf pediatric emergency cart in the recovery room where I work. On the top shelf is a fishing tackle box containing pediatric doses of emergency drugs, pediatric endotracheal tubes and equipment, I.V. catheters, and monitor electrodes. The other shelves contain small arm boards, diapers, blood pressure cuffs, and gowns. Face masks and oxygen tubing are kept in a cloth bag hung on the side of the cart.

When a pediatric patient is brought to the recovery room, we place the cart next to his bed. Then, if an emergency arises, we'll be prepared.

Deborah Stout, RN

Supportive measures

Familiar faces

Because most infants like to look at human faces, I cut faces out of magazines and securely attach them to cribs on our unit. And I ask the parents to bring in photographs of themselves. This way, family members get involved in the infant's care, and the infant feels more secure seeing familiar faces.

Wendy K. Pieri, RN, BSN

Allaying anxiety

To promote family bonding and ease parents' fears about their newborn's care, I make sure to involve the father—and when appropriate, the grandmother and other family members. For example, I ask the father to help bathe his newborn, comb her hair, and hold her hand during her first vitamin injection. The relatives are glad to support their new

baby and this practice improves my communication with the parents.

Wendy Kabiri, RN,C

Double banding

When you admit a pediatric patient who brings a favorite doll or stuffed animal with her, put an identification band on the toy (with the child's name on it) as well as on the child. This will make the child feel less alone. And it will ensure the prompt return of the toy to its owner if it should get lost.

V. Houck Vaira, RN

"Moon gas" medication

Here's how I help reduce a pediatric patient's fear and anxiety during an aerosol nebulizer treatment. I tell the child to pretend that he's an astronaut on a space mission and that the mask is a space mask. His goal is to withstand the "moon gas" (medication) so he can earn his flight wings. When the treatment is finished, I give him a sticker with a pair of wings on it.

Terrilynn M. Quillen, RN

From croup tent to castle

Trying to get a child to stay under a croup tent can be challenging. I make a game of it: I pretend the child is a prince (or princess) living in a castle. The child and I color pictures of windows and flags and tape them on the outside of the tent to make it look like a "castle." Then I cut out a paper crown with a number of tiers. We color in a jewel every time a "reward" is in order (such as when he takes his medication). I also give him safe toys to play with.

This way, he'll be preoccupied with the game and more inclined to stay under the tent.

Kara Watkins, RN, BSN

Sign on

When caring for young children with long-term tracheostomies, try teaching them sign language. This will not only make it easier for them to communicate with you, it will also promote language development and should help reduce the children's anxiety and frustration. Get the family and anyone else involved in their care to learn sign language, too.

Rhonda Quillin, RN

Sticker solution for pediatric patients

When I work in our pediatric unit, I carry sheets of decorative stickers to share with my patients. The stickers provide a diversion during examinations, and the children use them to decorate casts and large dressings—or themselves. They also provide a hard-to-miss spot to date dressings, tubing, and I.V. sites. I've even placed them on an anatomic dummy to help teach a preteen patient with diabetes how to rotate insulin injection sites.

Terrilynn Quillen, RN

Bubbles of fun

I've found a safe toy to keep a pediatric patient amused—bubbles.

You can make bubble liquid by mixing three parts liquid castile soap with one part water. A plastic piggyback I.V. hook works well as a wand. After dipping the wand in the liquid, the child can make bubbles by waving it in the air or by blowing on it. Bubbles are a great diversion during assessments and treatments, and they also encourage deep breathing. Of course, bubbles are appropriate only for older children who know not to drink the solution and who aren't in isolation. Also, someone should watch the children when they're using the bubbles.

Terrilynn M. Quillen, RN

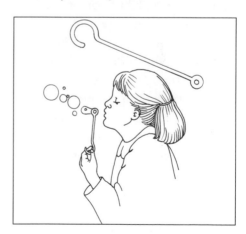

Helping kids face their fears

Pediatric patients who are in isolation won't be as frightened if you let them watch you put on your mask.

You might also draw a happy face on the mask to help soothe their fears.

Leslie A. Douglas, RN, MSN

Pediatric masquerade

To ease a hospitalized child's fear when he's placed in isolation, I use this approach. After explaining to the child and his family the purpose and techniques of isolation, I give the child his own paper gown and mask. I tell him he can use them to play "hospital" when he goes home. Besides arousing his interest, this reminds him that his stay is temporary.

Marsha Landfried, RN

A child's book

To minimize a child's fear of hospitalization and injury, try helping him create a book about his feelings. Encourage him to draw a picture each day that depicts how he feels. Ask him to explain the picture, then help him write a caption or story to go with it. Emphasize that the book is his to keep, but suggest that he might want to share it with his family.

You can "bind" the book by punching holes in the pages and tying them together with string.

Maun F. Hunsberger, RN

Pediatric exams: At the drawing table

I've found that a simple activity—drawing—helps to relieve a child's apprehension when he's waiting to see the doctor. So I leave a box of crayons for him to use on the white paper covering the examination table.

Marie Christopher, BSN

Out-of-sight I.V.

Pediatric patients seem to worry less when their I.V. lines are out of sight. So when we start a child's I.V., we secure it, then cover it with a cardboard paper towel roll that's been cut open lengthwise. We gently tape the roll to the child's arm. We also tape the ends of the cardboard for comfort and safety.

To check the I.V. site, we simply remove the roll, then replace it.

Louise Coull, RN

Cast covers for kids

A toddler with a broken arm may present a double challenge: how to keep his cast clean *and* in one piece. Here's an idea you can suggest to his parents.

Let the child pick out a piece of cotton material that he likes. Make a tube-shaped cover out of it, then sew a piece of elastic at each end so it will stay on the cast. This cover can be washed at the end of the day and used again.

Rebecca S. Renfro, RN

Trial run

During our preoperative teaching, we let children scheduled for short-stay elective surgery use a pediatric anesthesia mask. First, a nurse shows them how the mask works. Then each child tries the mask on and pretends to go to sleep for his operation. This reduces the children's fear and makes them much more cooperative.

Patricia McShane, RN

Teaching puppet

On our pediatric unit, we've learned the importance of preoperative teaching and try to use innovative approaches. For children scheduled to have tonsillectomies, we enlist the help of a puppet we call Herbie, who has removable tonsils. As we talk to the children about the procedure, we let them perform a tonsillectomy on Herbie. We use Herbie to help with postoperative instructions, too.

Donna Simpson, RN

Easing the fear of surgery

Surgery can be a frightening experience for a child, especially if he doesn't understand what's going on. So I've developed a "wound box" to help explain surgery.

First, I use a small box that opens on one side to represent the wound. Then, I place red felt inside to act as the muscle tissue. Blue ribbons are the blood vessels and a wad of white tissue paper is the fat. I also cut irregular shapes from fabric to represent general cellular growth. Finally, I cover the box with a knee-high stocking—the skin. It can be gathered to one side to demonstrate a suture line.

Marie Savoie, BSN

Give 'em a band

On our pediatric surgical unit, our patients *and* their favorite toys (teddy bears, dolls, or other security blankets) get identification bands. This way, we can quickly reunite the children with their toys after surgery, saving our young patients unnecessary emotional upset.

Mary Lu Rang, RN, BSN

Starred charts

When pediatric patients take their prescribed medications for the day, help them see stars. Stars on their medication charts, that is.

To make a chart, take a sheet of paper, print the patient's name on it, and list his prescribed medications down the left side. Then print the days of the week across the top of the page and add rules for the necessary columns. When the patient takes his medications, put an adhesive-backed star in that day's space. Giving stars as a reward really encourages patients to take their medications. And to encourage at-home compliance, give the chart to the child's parents when he leaves the hospital.

Brian J.J. Cole, SN

Schooltime sights

One of my duties as a school nurse is to test the vision of preschool children. Two problems in doing this are: (1) getting the child to stand at the correct distance from the eye chart; and (2) having him cover one eye without spreading his fingers and peeking.

To solve the first problem, I cut small feet patterns out of colored construction paper and tape them to the floor where the child should stand. He'll usually take great care to stand right on the paper feet during the vision test. To solve the second problem, I give the child a construction paper fish, which he holds by the tail so the fish's body covers his eye. No peeking now. After the test, the child can take the fish home.

Betty Hedlund, RN, BSN

Potential poisoning: Call for help first

I tell a child's parents to attach the phone numbers of their local poison control center and their pediatrician to a bottle of syrup of ipecac. These phone numbers are a reminder to contact the poison control center

before administering any treatment and to contact the pediatrician.

Terrilynn M. Quillen, RN

Handy notes for parents

When a new patient is admitted to our pediatric unit, we give his parents a handout with information on hospital policies, such as visiting hours and directions to the cafeteria. We add the names of the patient's doctor and primary nurse. This saves us time and keeps the parents informed.

Marcy Meitzner, RN

A new diagnostic tool: Lunch

When a child comes to the University of Illinois Hospital Affective Disorders Clinic for a 1-day evaluation, he and his parents are treated to lunch by a nursing staff member. But this "family luncheon" is more than just a social event. Conceived by doctors and carried out by the psychiatric clinical nurse specialist, it's also a diagnostic tool.

The informal luncheon is held in the hospital cafeteria or, if the weather's nice, in the hospital courtyard. While giving the child and parents a chance to meet with a member of the nursing staff away from the unit, the luncheon also lets the nurse see firsthand how the family interacts.

The result? The family feels more comfortable with the staff, who in turn gain greater insight into the child's problems.

After the luncheon, an assessment form documents the findings, which are shared with other staff members.

Janet York, RN, MSN

Replace your pin with paint

I use fabric paint to write my name and title on my own scrubs instead of wearing my identification pin, which can easily scratch a pediatric patient if dislodged.

Luann Collins, RN

Creating a smile

I give all of my pediatric patients a "Best Patient Award" certificate before they leave the busy outpatient surgery unit where I work. The certificate, which includes the patient's name, always makes children feel special and usually makes them smile. I created the certificate on our computer and the unit secretary prints one out for each patient.

Deborah Ashton, RN

5 HOME CARE

Medication reminder

A patient may forget a dose of a medication if he has a lot of tablets and capsules to take at different times of the day. One of my home-care patients has an easy way to remember, using a bulletin board. Here's what he does:

First he writes the times on separate pieces of paper and tacks them in chronological order across the top of the bulletin board. (Special instructions, such as "Take with plenty of water," could also be included.) Then he writes the days of the week vertically on the left-hand side of the board. Next, he fills self-sealing, plastic sandwich bags with the correct dose of medication for each specific time of day. (You or the patient may want to do this once a week.) Finally, he tacks the bag to the board under the appropriate day and time. He can tell at a glance when to take his medication, and he can see if he's forgotten a dose.

The bulletin board should be kept in a place where it is not accessible to children and should only be used if the patient is mentally alert. Also check to make sure that the medication will not be affected by exposure to light.

Karen Gray Pigott, RN

Egg-xact way to remember medications

As a home health care nurse, I've found that a patient may have difficulty opening a medicine bottle or knowing which medication to take next. An egg carton offers a simple solution.

Label each pocket of the carton with the dosage schedule in consecutive order for 1 day. Then place the proper medication into the corresponding pocket. The cartons can be stacked so that a family member or friend can prepare medications for several days at one time.

Of course, remind the patient to keep the cartons out of the reach of children.

Leslie M. Attig, RN

Eggsactly the right dose

A big problem for a patient who's discharged with a lot of medications is how to adjust his hospital medication schedule to his at-home schedule. To help him, I review *both* schedules with the patient before he's discharged.

First, we discuss the patient's normal routine at home, for example, when he wakes, eats, sleeps, and so on. With this routine in mind, we list the times it would be convenient and appropriate for him to take his medications. To make it easier, we try to group medications by scheduling the b.i.d. doses for the same time as two of the q.i.d. doses.

Using an egg carton, we mark one of these times in front of one of the depressions in the front row. Then we mark another medication time in front of the next depression, and so on until all of the medication times have been marked on the egg carton. We place the medication containers in the second row.

Each night at home, the patient sets up his next day's medications in the egg carton. Taking one container at a time from the second row, he removes the medications and places them in the appropriately marked time depressions in the first row. The next day, he just takes his medications at the times marked on the carton. He doesn't have to worry about double or missed doses.

Tell your patient to keep the egg carton out of the sunlight and out of the reach of children. And if you're worried about the medications' exposure to room air and moisture, check with the patient's doctor or pharmacist before setting up the system.

Anna Juskiw, RN, BS

Keeping *track* of medications

When a patient needs to take several medications every day, suggest that he arrange his pill bottles in an empty spice rack. Each shelf should be labeled according to the time of day he takes each pill (morning, noon, or evening). For medications taken more than once a day, he can move the bottle to the next appropriate shelf after he takes each dose.

Remind him to keep the rack out of the reach of children.

Joan Jimerson, RN

Handy hankie

Here's a nifty way to teach patients to keep their nitroglycerin tablets handy at all times. Place the bottle of tablets in the center of an open handkerchief. Fold the four corners around the bottle. Then pierce the corners with a safety pin and attach the handkerchief to the patient's clothing. The patient can remove the bottle without unpinning the handkerchief by simply slipping it through one of the side holes.

Tara Hummel, RN,C

Safe storage for nitroglycerin tablets

An elderly person may have trouble keeping track of his nitroglycerin tablets. Here's a way to make a convenient and safe storage place for them:

He should make two vertical slits in one side of an old 35-mm film canister. (You can do this for him if he can't.) These slits will allow him to slide the container onto his belt. Then he can place the bottle of nitroglycerin tablets into the container and replace the lid.

Robert N. Anderson, RN, CCRN, CEN

Right side up—and down

Do your patients on twice-daily medications have trouble remembering whether they've taken their morning or evening dose? Here's a way to help them keep track:

Tell them to mark the top of the medication container "a.m." and the bottom "p.m." Then, as soon as they've taken the medication, they can turn the container to show the time for the next dose. Later, if they've forgotten whether they took their medicine that morning, they can simply look at the contain

er. If it shows "p.m.," they know they took the morning dose.

Wilhelmina K. Patterson, RN

A feeling for healing

A pharmacist came up with this idea to help a blind patient identify the different medications he had to take at home every day. He devised a code using letters and simple symbols to represent the medications and times they were to be taken.

For example, a triangle (3 sides) represents t.i.d.; a square (4 sides), q.i.d.; and a letter of the alphabet, the name of the medication. He cut these letters and symbols out of carpet tape and attached them to the appropriate bottles. The patient could "read" these labels, using his sense of touch.

Sylvia T. Joseph, RN

Taking medication: Help for the blind

When I was caring for a blind woman who had to take multiple medications, I wanted to do something to help her become more independent. So I decided to customize each medication bottle.

I went to the pharmacy and got medication bottles without child-proof caps. Next, I asked the recreational therapist for some raised shapes. I placed one shape on each of the bottles and on each of the lids, along with the name of the drug in the bottle. Then I tape-recorded her medication schedule, including the name of each drug, when to take it, and the shape on the corresponding lid.

Janet Paluck, RN

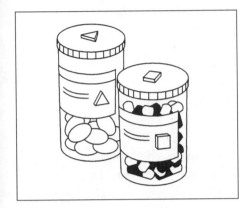

Easy-to-find insulin

When I work with diabetic home health care patients who can't read or who have poor eyesight, I prefill their insulin syringes and put them in familiar containers. For example, I'll put morning doses in a coffee can and label the can "morning" in big letters and put evening doses in a vegetable bin and label it "evening."

Phyllis Houchens, RN

Bottle clip

A simple, inexpensive broom clip holder helps a one-handed diabetic patient prepare his insulin independently.

The clip, available in most hardware stores, holds a standard-size insulin bottle securely and can be mounted onto any convenient surface with a single screw. An easy-to-reach kitchen cabinet shelf usually works well. (Of course, the clip shouldn't interfere with closing the cabinet door.)

June B. Jackson, OTR

Using the right syringe at the right time

Sometimes I have to prefill insulin syringes for one of my home health care patients because he has poor coordination. To help him identify his morning and evening doses, I place the morning syringes in a yellow cup on the top shelf of his refrigerator and the evening syringes in a black cup on the bottom shelf. The yellow on top will remind him that this is his morning dose; the black on the bottom signals his night dose.

This method is easy to remember, and it reassures the patient that he's using the right syringe at the right time.

Marion Jackel Wilson, LPN

Sharps safety

I tell my diabetic patients to dispose of used lancets and syringes in an empty, plastic laundry detergent bottle. After the bottle is about three-quarters full, I suggest that the patient pour plaster of Paris into it. Once the mixture hardens, he can place the container in the trash.

Cynthia Mik, RN, CDE

Dispense with ease

Patients who have arthritis or can use only one hand may have trouble pouring liquids from containers. Instead of struggling, they can ask a family member to pour the liquids into pump dispensers. These dispensers are available in large sizes for beverages and in small sizes for condiments, lotion, and shampoo.

Terrilynn M. Quillen, RN

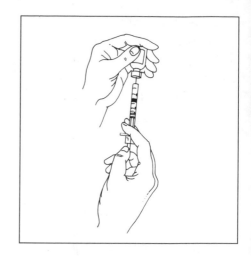

Add color for clarity

My home health care patient's wife wasn't sure she was giving her husband the right dose of oral morphine. Because it's a clear solution, it was difficult to tell when she'd reached the correct line on the scored dropper.

After checking with a pharmacist, I told her to add two drops of red food coloring to the morphine. Now she can see the level clearly, and she isn't worried about giving the wrong dose.

Lois Schlabsz, RN

A drop in the eyeglass

When my husband had trouble instilling his eyedrops after eye surgery, I came up with a simple solution. I took a pair of inexpensive plastic sunglasses (polarized glasses won't work) and made a hole in the middle of each lens, using a large-bore needle. My husband put on the glasses and instilled the drops through the holes. Of course, I made sure that he kept the glasses and dropper clean.

Joanne Curtin, RN

Liquid meds: Line of demarcation

A home health care patient can make sure he's drawing up the correct amount of liquid medication by marking the syringe's fill line with red nail polish. That way, he'll know how far to fill the syringe—even if the numbers wear off.

Connie Sarvis, RN, BN, MN

Keeping track of flushed lumens

I've found a way to teach a home health care patient how to ensure that he's flushed all the lumens of his multiple-lumen central venous catheter. After we prepare the correct number of flushes, the patient and I decide how to refer to the flushing sequence of the lumens, such as left to right or shortest to longest. If the patient loses track of which lumens he flushed, he can count the flushes he has left and immediately know which lumen to flush next.

Sheila Ledermann, RN

Fostering independence

Ready resource for home-bound patients

During my initial home health care visit, I give the patient an emergency sheet that lists my agency's daytime and after-hours phone numbers in large, bold print at the top and bottom of the paper. It also lists the nursing specialties the agency offers, the names of the specialty nurses, and the name and phone number of the patient's doctor. Posted on the refrigerator or near the phone, this sheet is a ready resource for a patient and his family.

Leah McNulty, RN, BSN

A pencil pusher

In the large nursing home where I work, some wheelchair patients couldn't reach the elevator's 8th-floor button. So I suggested they carry a new, unsharpened pencil with them and use the rubber eraser to press the button.

The pencil adds almost 4" to their reach and gives them a new feeling of independence. Now they don't have to wait until someone has time to take them to their 8th-floor rooms or activities—they just reach up and go themselves.

Catherine Barnshaw, LPN

Improved walker

Help a patient with a walker become more independent and surefooted by buying a bicycle basket and attaching it to the front of his walker. He can then go to stores by himself and carry his packages home in the basket. And he'll become much steadier, thanks to the increased practice and exercise.

Suzanne Devine, RN

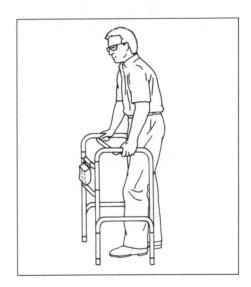

Smoother transport

After he's discharged, a patient with limited mobility may have trouble carrying things. A few household items may come in handy.

He can clip a pet leash to a filled laundry basket and drag the basket across the floor. Or he can put things on a rolling plant stand and push the stand from room to room. And a small wagon is great for moving heavier items.

Terrilynn Quillen, RN

Stuck-up cane

A friend who has multiple sclerosis and uses a cane passed along this tip to me. Whenever he'd lean his cane against a wall or counter to free both his hands, the cane would invariably drop to the floor. Retrieving it was always a struggle.

To solve this problem, he attached a small piece of Velcro to the handle of his cane and attached matching pieces to his belt, workbench, filing cabinet, kitchen counter, and wherever else he usually propped his cane. Now whenever he has to use both hands, he "hangs" his cane on the Velcro, and it stays upright until he needs it again.

Ann T. Nandrea, RN

Leg lifts

After he goes home, a patient who has a knee or leg cast can try this technique for getting out of bed: Put the collar end of a dog leash around the lower part of the leg that's in the cast. Hold the other end of the leash and swing the leg out of bed.

Debby Newton, RN

Working on the rails

I recently cared for a patient in his home who spent most of the time in bed. Whenever he tried to raise himself, he'd have trouble holding onto the slippery bed rails.

To help, I bought two 3' pieces of formed foam rubber from a hardware store (they're usually wrapped around hot water pipes for insulation). I wrapped the pieces around the bed rails and taped them in place.

The foam rubber rail pads are inexpensive. They've been in place for more than 4 months and still look fine. Best of all, they do the job: they give the patient a sure grip whenever he wants to lift himself in bed.

Ethel Hamilton, LPN

Seeds of contentment

One of my home care patients recently confided to me that he was bored with his daily routine of reading and watching television. During our conversation, I discovered that he was a bird lover. I asked a family member to mount a board on the sill outside his bedroom window and to put some birdseed on the board. Now many different birds make a habit of helping themselves to the birdseed, and my patient spends a pleasant hour or so every day observing and identifying them.

Theresa Tucker, RN

Soap on a rope

A home health care patient with limited mobility may have trouble using soap and a washcloth in the shower. Here's a way to solve the problem:

Put the bar of soap in the leg of an old pair of panty hose. Knot the panty hose above and below the bar to form a loop; then hang the soap on a shower rack or chair from this loop.

Now the patient can reach the soap without having to bend over and risk falling. The nylon allows him to grip the soap. And because the nylon is mildly abrasive, he doesn't need a washcloth.

Terrilynn Quillen, RN

No more bath blues

If a rheumatoid arthritis patient can't bathe himself, use a special bath sponge and heavy wire coat hanger. Stretch the top and bottom of the hanger. At the bottom, shape a triangle, stitch a folded sponge around it, and then fold a washcloth around the sponge. Adjust the hook at the top for the patient's best grip and bend the handle to suit his washing needs. If his elbows or wrists are too stiff to use the device, he could bend the handle into another position.

And how can a patient with stiff fingers squeeze out the sponge and cloth? If he places the sponge against the side of the basin, he can press his hand flat against the sponge.

Louise Wiedmer, RN

Using a mirror for central line care

When he returns home, a patient may find that dressing changes are the most frustrating part of central line care. So before he's discharged, I tell him to use a mirror when he changes a dressing. (A small compact or makeup mirror works well.) The mirror will help him see what he's doing and allow him to check the site for signs of infection.

Beverly A. Anderson, RN,C, ONC, MS

Lace-free shoes

A person with arthritis may have trouble lacing his shoes. You can help him solve this frustrating problem by replacing the laces with $\frac{1}{4}$"-wide elastic. Because the elastic stretches, putting the shoes on or taking them off will be a snap. You should also remind him to check the elastic periodically to make sure it's not too tight.

Marie M. Savoie, BSN

Brush up on fun

Some elderly patients in nursing homes and those who have arthritis or paralysis may be missing out on some fun because they can't hold playing cards or magazines. To help them participate in such activities, give them a scrub brush. With the bristle end up, the brush can hold cards, pictures, and even light magazines.

Linda Jeronovitz, RN

Improvising equipment

Homemade strainer

Coffee filters and ordinary collection cups are inexpensive alternatives to medical-grade strainer-collectors for home health care patients who must strain urine for stones. Coffee filters can even collect the tinier stones that sometimes pass through the plastic mesh of traditional collection units.

Terrilynn Quillen, RN

Slow-cooker compresses

If my home health care patient needs warm compresses, I keep them in his room in an uncovered slow-cooker set on the lowest temperature. That way, they're always ready for use. I check the slow-cooker periodically to make sure it doesn't get too hot and review precautions with my patient before he does this on his own.

Wanda Denson, LVN

Alternative ice pack

When a patient is going home, I give him this simple tip for a homemade ice pack: If he doesn't have a regular ice pack, but he does have a 16-oz bag of frozen peas on hand, he can place the peas in a pillowcase. Then he'll have an inexpensive, versatile substitute that won't leak. The peas can be refrozen for repeated use. Remind him to mark the bag so he doesn't inadvertently cook and con-

sume his ice pack.

Cory McKeown, RN

Do-it-yourself ice pack

Tell your patients who need to apply ice to an injury at home to make their own ice packs instead of buying expensive ones. Here's what they'll need to do. Pour 3 cups of water and 1 cup of rubbing alcohol into a plastic resealable bag. Seal the bag, place it inside another bag, and put it in the freezer for 8 to 12 hours. The pack won't freeze solid, but will have a soft, gel-like consistency that molds to any body area.

Terri Lynn Gross, RN

Freezer wrap

For the patient who needs to continue cryogenic therapy at home, suggest that he make a quick and easy ice pack. Here's how:

Wrap a wet towel around a coffee can and put it in the freezer. After the towel freezes, remove it from the can and wrap it around the injured area. Cover the towel loosely with an elastic bandage to hold it in place and prevent it from leaking.

Wayne D. McDowell, RN

Heavy chairs for rails

When patients return home after surgery, they may miss using those hospital bed side rails to turn and get out of bed. If they have this problem, suggest that they put a *heavy* chair that won't tip over next to the bed. They can use the arm or the back of the chair as a "rail" when they want to turn or get up.

Make sure you point out that the chair must be heavy enough to withstand pushing and pulling. Putting something on the chair seat will make it even more stable.

Michelle A. Crumrine, RN

Elevating idea

For a home care patient who doesn't have a hospital bed but needs to elevate his head or leg, try this: Place one or more pillows under the mattress at the end of the bed that needs to be raised. Placing the pillows under the mattress instead of on top of it will prevent them from moving when the patient turns.

Mary Boutcher, RN, DON

Fluffing up a foam mattress

Here's an easy home health care tip: If a convoluted foam mattress flattens in the middle, you can revive it

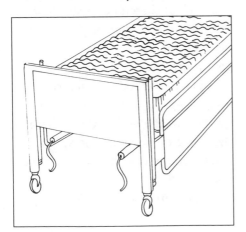

by using a hand-held blow dryer. Set the dryer on high and hold it 1" to 2" from the flattened cones. The heat and air from the dryer will fluff them within a few minutes.

Laurie Gailunas, LPN

Bed 'n' board ('n' bag 'n' books)

Bedridden patients sometimes need the head of their bed raised for comfort. With a hospital bed, this is no problem. To raise a regular bed, though, you might suggest they try one of the following:

• Wedge a beanbag chair between the mattress and box spring. The chair will raise the head of the bed about 30 degrees. (Before doing this, though, the patient should check with the mattress manufacturer to make sure that bending it at this angle won't damage it.)

• Put a few boards or books under the legs at the head of the bed.

• Slant a wide board (or a few boards) from the middle of the bed to the top of the headboard. Then tie the boards to the headboard and bed to keep them in place, and pad the boards with sheets, blankets, and pillows.

Whatever method the patient chooses, he'll have the comfort of a hospital bed without the expense.

Ann McCormick, RN, CCRN

Bed board

To set up a large table for patients confined to bed at home, try using an adjustable ironing board. Just position it across the bed, adjust the height, and the patient will have room to keep books and papers and even to eat meals.

Lorie Alwes, LPN, NA

A pull sheet

One of my elderly home care patients is a big man who's too debilitated to pull himself up in bed. His wife, a small woman, isn't strong enough to pull him up either. With a little ingenuity and teamwork, though, they discovered a way to move him.

They twisted a flat bed sheet into a rope and placed it across the bed, under the patient's shoulders. They brought the ends of the sheet under his armpits, over his shoulders, and over the head of the bed. Then the wife grips each end and, with the patient pushing with his feet, she can pull him up in bed.

Pam Barton, RN

Custom gown: Quick cut

Here's an easy way for a family member to make a gown for a home health care patient: Have the family member cut a cotton nightgown up the back and hem the edges so that they don't fray. The result is a gown that works great for a bedridden patient, especially if he's incontinent.

Leah McNulty, RN, BSN

Padded socks

An elderly home care patient wanted some elbow protectors. I didn't have any with me, so I suggested she make them herself.

I told her to cut the tops and toes off an old pair of socks. She could then place a sanitary pad (with an adhesive strip) inside each sock, lengthwise over the heel. This makes a pair of comfortable, inexpensive elbow (or heel) protectors.

Angelina Elkin, RN

Enterprising idea

As a home health care nurse, I sometimes have to improvise procedures. I once used this technique to administer an enema to an elderly patient who didn't have the necessary supplies. I positioned the patient on a rubber pad on her left side with her right knee drawn up to her chest. Then I lubricated about 6" of the end of a sterile #16 French catheter with K-Y jelly and inserted the catheter slowly and gently into the patient's rectum.

Next, I attached a 60-ml irrigating syringe filled with the enema solution to the end of the catheter. By raising or lowering the syringe, I could control the flow of water into the rectum.

Barbara Malcomb, RN, PHN

Dental assistant

Here's a tip to pass on to postoperative dental patients: If bleeding occurs at home, and the patient has no gauze on hand, he can use a tampon instead. Tell him to just cut the tampon in half, place one half at the bleeding site and bite down. This will stanch the bleeding and save a phone call to the dentist.

Lynne Cole, RN

Postpartum pads

If your postpartum patient is breastfeeding her baby, she may appreciate this tip:

Instead of commercial bra pads, try using beltless sanitary minipads. Simply cut a minipad in half, peel the backing off both halves, and affix one half to each side of the bra.

The minipad halves are highly absorbent and have a stay-dry lining that helps prevent irritated nipples and leaking. Besides, they're much cheaper—less than half the cost of most commercial bra pads.

Susan Lea, RN
Marie M. Savoie, BSN

Padded protection for wet wound

After my husband's hemorrhoidectomy, he was given gauze to protect his briefs from postoperative bleeding. He complained that the gauze was bulky and slipped around; I was concerned because it stayed moist with blood, increasing the risk of infection to the incision.

I suggested he use unscented, self-adhering minipads instead of the gauze. The pads stayed in place and their absorbent inner layer kept the area dry. (They can probably be used after other types of rectal surgery, too.)

Sheryl Stone Clay, RN, BSN

Reflections on wounds

After being hospitalized for abdominal surgery, I was sent home with instructions to clean and redress the wound. To accomplish this, I improvised the following method:

I put a disposable underpad on my bed and arranged all the necessary supplies nearby. Then I lay down on the bed with two pillows under my shoulders and head, knees flexed, and a hand mirror propped against them. This way I could see the wound and use both hands for the cleaning and dressing change.

Donna M. Babao, RN, MA

Protective padding

I encourage my home health care patients who require dressing changes to buy a diaper-changing pad. This way, their dressings can be changed on top of the pad, using the nonabsorbent side to protect bed linens and the padded side to cushion the wound during the procedure. Tell the patient or his caregiver to wash the pad daily and wipe it with an antiseptic after each use.

Carla Goodmurphy, RN, OCN

I.V. supplies: In the bag

A home health care patient requiring routine I.V. fluids can store his I.V. supplies in a clear vinyl, multipocket, over-the-door shoe bag. The bag takes up little space and the vinyl, which is easy to disinfect, allows the patient to see exactly where everything is. The bag is also convenient for traveling; the patient can just take it off the door, roll it up, then unroll and hang it when he gets where he's going. Make sure you tell your patient to keep the bag away from children.

Terrilynn Quillen, RN

Weathering home infusion

I care for outpatients who require portable infusion pumps to administer continuous chemotherapy. When a snowstorm is on the way, I send each of these patients home with a flush kit. In the kit, I include a 10-ml normal saline solution flush, a 5-ml heparin flush, alcohol pads, safety gloves, absorbent pads, gauze pads, and a resealable bag. I teach the patient how to safely disconnect the pump and flush the venous access device at home after the infusion is finished. This way, he can maintain catheter patency and prevent complications until he can safely return to the hospital.

Colleen A. Carey, RN, BSN

Bath apron: If the bag fits...

If you're caring for a patient in his home, you'll need a bath apron. You can make your own from a hanging shoe bag.

First, remove the metal pieces from the vinyl bag. Secure one end of a piece of woven tape, rope, or cord to the upper left-hand corner and the other end to the upper right-hand corner. This makes a loop that will fit around your neck and hold the bag in place. Attach a piece of cord to each side to tie the bag around your waist.

These bags have several compartments, so you can take everything you need into the bathroom. The vinyl cleans easily, and it will keep your uniform dry during the patient's bath.

Terrilynn Quillen, RN

Face saver

One of my home health care patients has arthritis, and when I wash her hair in the shower, she can't tilt her head back to keep the water and shampoo from getting into her eyes and ears. To help her, I cut a big circle out of the top of a plastic shower cap. I put the cap on her head, pulling her hair through the cut-out circle. The elastic rim is now above her eyes and ears, so I simply flip down the remaining plastic to protect her face.

Now she doesn't have to move

her head at all, and she doesn't get any water or shampoo in her eyes or ears either.

Ruth Sagehorn, RN

Support board for legs

Most wheelchairs don't have enough support for a patient who needs to keep his leg elevated. To solve this problem, several staff members designed a support board to fit across the chair's elevated leg rests. Here's how you can make your own:

Cut a piece of 1"-thick plywood 2" longer than the width of the wheelchair. Place foam that's at least 2" thick over the board; then cover with vinyl material. Attach reclosable straps to either end of the board. These straps will secure the board to the leg rests.

A board can be made to fit any wheelchair. It provides secure support even for a leg that's in a cast, and it can be easily cleaned and disinfected if necessary.

Roslyn M. Gleeson, RN,C, MSN

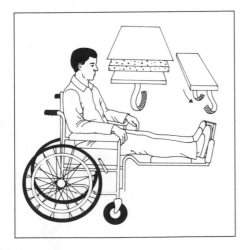

Lighter load

Because patients with back problems shouldn't carry anything heavy, I suggest that they use a luggage carrier to tote heavy packages. This will allow them to continue their daily routine and still comply with discharge instructions.

Shelley Carlson, RN

Humidity hang-up

To increase the humidity in a home care patient's room without a humidifier, just hang a damp bath towel over a vinyl- or plastic-covered chair and place the chair near the radiator or baseboard. As the towel dries, the room air quickly becomes moist—even more quickly, it seems, than it would if you placed a pan of water near the heat.

Audrey Gilmore, RN,C

Tackling organization

As a home health care nurse, I use a tackle box to keep my venipuncture supplies organized. The box's small compartments and carrying handle are great conveniences.

Angie Perry, RN

DISK-advantage

As a home health care nurse, I frequently need more equipment than I like to carry with me. For instance, when measuring the size of lesions or decubitus ulcers, I find the tip of my finger not exact enough but rulers too bulky *and* breakable.

My solution is to carry a measurement disk made for reading the results of intradermal skin tests. It's accurate and easy to carry. If the disks aren't available at the home health agency, I can get a supply simply by writing to the drug companies that manufacture the skin tests.

Jill Dailer, RN, BSN

Resolving elimination

Protecting skin with a sock
A patient with a urinary leg bag may develop skin rashes and excoriation, especially in warm weather. Here's how I make him more comfortable.

I cut off the foot of a tube sock and pull the sock over the patient's knee to midthigh; I make sure the sock isn't too tight. The bag rests against the sock—which protects his skin—and is secured with the leg strap. The sock is easy to keep clean, and it absorbs perspiration.

Kathy Tweed, LPN

Preventing urine backflow
If your patient is discharged with a urinary catheter, tell him to hang the drainage bag from a mattress handle at night. This will secure the bag below his bladder, preventing urine backflow while he's sleeping. If his drainage bag can't be hooked, advise him to place it in a recyclable plastic shopping bag and tie the shopping bag around one of the mattress handles. If his mattress doesn't have handles, tell him to place the drainage bag in a large plastic bag and tuck the opening well under the mattress so that the bag dangles down.

Angie Fuller, RN, BSN

Expedient extract
Liquids and tablets for deodorizing ostomy appliances are sometimes expensive and ineffective. Vanilla extract is an effective and inexpensive alternative. Instruct patients to saturate a small wad of tissue with vanilla extract and place it in the bottom of the appliance. They can repeat this procedure as often as necessary—every time they empty the appliance, if they desire.

Diane Deegan-McCrann, RN, ET

Cleaning on the go
Cleaning a colostomy or ileostomy pouch can be difficult for a home health care patient. I suggest he purchase a small plastic squeeze bottle (they are inexpensive and available at any drugstore) that has a screw-on top. He can carry the bottle in his jacket pocket and fill it with tap water when needed. This way he'll be able to keep the pouch clean, no matter where he is.

Donna Eichna, RN, CS, MSN

Odor-free colostomy care
To reduce the odor from a colostomy bag when you empty and rinse it, add some mouthwash to the

water you use to rinse the bag. Put a small amount of mouthwash in the bag before you close it, too.

Share this tip with the patient's family to make colostomy care easier for everyone.

Joan Woods, RN

Colostomy cleanup

Here's a tip for your patient with a colostomy: Suggest he spray the inside of his colostomy bag with a cooking oil spray before applying the bag. His stools won't stick to the bag, and cleanup will be easier.

Teresa Ryan, RN

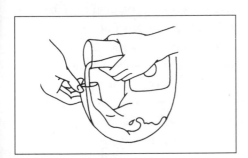

Better than a bedpan

As a home hospice nurse, I've found that female patients often prefer female urinals to bedpans. The urinals are inexpensive and easier to use.

JoAnn Shenk, BSN

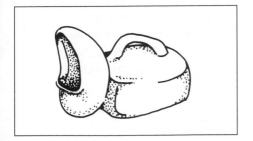

Substitute straps

One of my elderly home care patients had an indwelling urinary catheter with a leg bag. The straps on the bag dug into his skin, causing irritation. In looking for substitute straps for the bag, I noticed the strap on a Depend adult disposable undergarment. This strap is wide and stretchy, and it has two buttons on each end. I wrapped the strap around the patient's leg and attached the leg bag to the buttons. The strap stays in place and doesn't harm the patient's skin.

Margaret Guilfoyle, RN

Nighttime convenience

One of my home care patients has nurses assigned to her in the day and evening but not at night. Urinary frequency is a problem because she can't get out of bed to go to the bathroom without someone helping her. So before the evening nurse leaves, she puts a bedpan on top of a bucket near the patient's bed. During the night, the patient can reach over, get the bedpan, use it, and empty it into the bucket. She can reuse the bedpan as often as necessary without worrying about spilling.

Pauline Lamia, RN

A filter tip

Here's a tip for your patients who must strain their urine for renal calculi or gravel. A cone-shaped filter for an automatic coffee maker makes a handy urine strainer. The filters are small-pored and can be easily handled and disposed of. Also, if the patient passes any blood that's not readily visible, a pink or red stain will appear on the white filter paper.

Arline M. Brice, SN

Imaginative laxative

Try making this "milk shake" for constipated patients who won't drink prune juice. Mix ice cream with the juice and blend to drinking consistency.

Patti Nielsen, RN

Solving intake problems

Tracking fluid flow

To help my fluid-restricted home health care patient keep track of his fluid intake, I tell him to put an empty quart container in the kitchen each morning. (If your patient is allowed a different amount of fluid, mark the container accordingly or use one of a different size.) Every time he takes a drink, he pours an equal amount of fluid into the container. When the container is full, he knows he's had his limit.

Melissa Gilliland, RN

To a tee

Surgical patients discharged with a long-term or permanent feeding tube, which must be clamped between feedings to prevent backflow, sometimes lose the clamp and are unable to find a replacement. A plastic or wooden golf tee is a readily available substitute that fits perfectly into the end of a nasogastric tube.

D. Peters, RN

Cool food in hot weather

During the hot summer months, a home care patient's enteral feeding bag may not stay cool enough. If that's a problem, slip the feeding bag and a frozen cold pack (the kind used in coolers for picnics) into a plastic storage bag. Punch a hole in the storage bag, about 2" up, for the feeding tube. Then wrap the bag in a towel to absorb condensation.

This will reduce the risk of bacterial growth in the enteral food.

Elaine A. Peterson, RN

Well-oiled

Many of my home care patients who receive frequent gastrostomy tube feedings find that the plungers of their 60-ml syringes become stiff and difficult to slide into the barrel of the syringe. To make the syringes easier to insert, I advise my patients to dip the tip of the plunger in vegetable oil before each feeding. Then the plunger will slide with ease.

Patricia Maskell, RN, BSN

Improving physical care

Diminutive dressing

Here's a suggestion for postoperative patients who need just a small dressing or protective cover for their incision when they're discharged: Apply a sanitary pad with an adhesive strip to the undergarment covering the incision. The pad protects the incision, is more economical than a sterile dressing, and has no adhesive touching the skin to irritate the sensitive surgical site (the adhesive strip is attached to the garment).

Carol I. Lewis, RN

Preheated veins

I frequently need to collect blood specimens from our home care patients, but many of them have poor veins for venipunctures. To save the time and discomfort of repeated needle sticks, I call the patient's home about 20 minutes before I'm scheduled to visit there. I tell the patient or a family member to apply a warm compress over the patient's inner arm at the elbow (the antecubital area). First, apply a warm, wet cloth; cover it with a dry cloth and put plastic wrap around the arm; and leave this compress in place until I arrive.

When I remove the compress from the patient's arm, his veins are more visible and easy to dilate, so the venipuncture is usually successful the first time around.

P. Stilger, RN

Taking off a tick

With summer approaching, we know we'll receive many inquiries in our emergency department about how to remove ticks. We recommend putting nail polish on the tick or touching its body with a warm match. Either way, the tick will pull its body out of the skin.

This is much easier than trying to remove the tick with tweezers. The tweezers might tear the tick, so some of its body would still be in the skin.

Polly Zimmermann, RN, BS

Finger splinting good

In an emergency, a hollow roller-type hair curler or the top half of the clamp-on curler will make a sturdy finger splint or protector for an injured finger.

Kathleen Cruzic

Kitchen cream

Since diabetic patients need to take special care of their feet, tell them they probably have an effective, inexpensive cream right in their own kitchen that will help soften their dry, calloused skin. It's solid vegetable shortening.

Tell the diabetic patient to put a dab of shortening in the palm of his hand after bathing. Then have him add a few drops of water and mix with the shortening until he gets a nice cream that rubs in well and doesn't leave a greasy covering. Using this treatment once or twice a day will bring dramatic results.

What's more, the "cream" can be used on elbows, hands, knees—wherever rough skin is a problem.

Joyce A. McCarthy, RN

Summer skin: Beating the heat

Summer's heat and humidity can cause irritation and moisture in a patient's skin folds. So I tell my home health care patients to dry carefully after bathing and then use a light dusting of cornstarch. I also suggest using antiperspirant in these skin folds, although I caution them never to apply it to broken or irritated areas.

Mary J. O'Donnell, RN

Soothing itchy skin—on the cheap

Oatmeal-based bath packets are effective in relieving pruritus from chickenpox and poison ivy, but they're expensive. My alternative:

I place ½ to ¼ cup of quick-cooking raw oatmeal in a cotton sock. Then I saturate and wring out the sock under the bathtub spout as the tub is filling with water. The oatmeal sock makes the bath water as soothing as a bath packet would,

and at a much lower price.

Sheryl Stone Clay, RN, BSN

Ostomy wafers: Preventing perspiration

Tell your ostomy patient to wipe his skin with a 5-day deodorant pad before applying an ostomy wafer. This will help control perspiration and prevent the wafer from loosening. He'll also save money because he won't need to change his appliance as often.

Joan Jacoby, RN

Skin debridement at home

If your home health care patient has a hand-held shower head, he can debride a leg ulcer himself. Here's how:

Tell the patient to hold the nozzle of the shower head about 6" from his ulcer and run warm water over it for 5 minutes. (If he has a shower chair, he might want to sit on it for comfort.)

He should do this twice a day until his ulcer heals. Of course, he should discontinue treatment if it causes pain.

Marion B. Dolan, RN

Coded clothes

An elderly, blind woman who lives alone recently told me how she coordinates the colors in her wardrobe: She uses safety pins to code the clothing by color. For instance, one pin placed on a garment in a vertical position indicates that the garment is white. Two vertical pins indicate that the garment is blue. Pins placed horizontally indicate other colors.

The coding system helps the woman retain her independence because it allows her to dress properly without assistance.

Carol Taylor, RN, MSN

Leg writing

When I discovered that my postoperative patients who'd had cesarean sections weren't doing their leg rotations and flexions in bed, I came up with another exercise routine. I asked them to pretend each leg is a pencil. They are to lift their "pencils" (one leg at a time) and print their newborn's *full* name in the air. No shortcuts with nicknames are allowed.

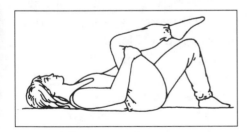

Now my patients are more compliant and even do their exercises more frequently.

Rita A. Bednarczyk, LPN

Home care helper

When a bedridden, chronically ill patient goes home, encourage his family members to buy or rent an inexpensive, portable intercom and place it in his bedroom. This will allow them to go into other areas of the house and still know when their loved one needs care.

Lynn Nelson, RN

Calling cards

When I was a home health care nurse, I found that patients often forgot scheduled appointment times and so weren't home when I arrived.

To avoid this, I started giving each patient my business card with his next appointment written on the back. Besides having the reminder, he also had the agency's phone number handy if he needed to call.

Jill Dailer, RN, BSN

Video tips for home-care nurses

At our home health care agency, we use videocassette tapes about patients whose care may be especially difficult. When a nurse has a new assignment, she can view the tape and pick up hints for the best way to handle her patient.

Joann Walbrecker, RN

Travel tips

In the can

A diabetic patient can carry an insulin bottle and two alcohol wipes in a 35-mm film canister. The canister allows a patient to take his insulin with him wherever he goes, without worrying about leakage or breakage.

Sue Ingram, RN

Injectable drugs to go

A toothbrush holder is a convenient, safe way to carry an injectable drug. The tube-shaped holder can accommodate a filled syringe, alcohol wipe, and bandage.

Connie Williams, LPN

Smooth entry

Here's an idea you might want to share with the families of arthritic patients:

To help a patient with arthritis get in and out of a car, cover the car seat with two sheets of heavy plastic. Tuck in the first sheet of plastic so it won't move, then place the second sheet on top of it. (Leave this second sheet loose.) The top sheet will slide against the bottom one, allowing the patient to enter the car smoothly.

I tried this with my arthritic grandmother, who's now getting in and out of my car twice as fast as before.

Donna A. Milner, LPN

Shopping bag for wheelchair patients

A different kind of shopping bag can make trips to the mall safer and more enjoyable for families of patients who require a wheelchair. Suggest that they buy a large, zippered, plastic pillow cover. With bias binding or hem tape, they can sew a loop on each side of the pillow cover, near the opening. The loops should fit onto the wheelchair handles. The bag, hanging behind the chair, will hold many packages.

I made a bag like this 7 years ago for my daughter's wheelchair, and it has worked well for us.

Dorothy I. Lissenden, RN

Hooked on hangers

Wire coat hangers work great as bag hooks for I.V. or enteral feeding solutions. So I advise my home health care patients with I.V. lines or enteral feeding tubes to take hangers with them on vacation. The hangers can be bent into bag hooks and then hung over doorways, closet bars, or picture frames.

Marion Casey Renz, RN, BS

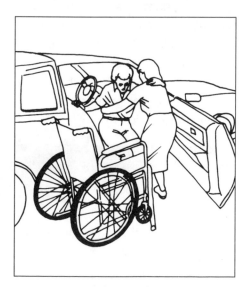

Quick fix for stoma leaks

Stoma patients may worry about what to do if their pouches or sites leak, so show them how to prepare an emergency kit. The contents are a pair of underpants, a stoma bag, a small facecloth or premoistened towelettes, and a small, plastic bottle of deodorant.

Men can put all this in a shaving kit; women can fit it in a makeup kit. Then the kit can be placed in a glove compartment or desk drawer, where it will be readily available, yet not arouse anyone's curiosity.

Jean Bourgelais, RN, ET

Marked map

As a home care nurse, I sometimes have trouble finding a patient's address when I'm unfamiliar with the area. So I cut a city map into 8" x 12" sections. I put two sections back to back, covering both sides with plastic and sealing the edges. Each morning, I draw my route in erasable marker on the plastic-coated map. This provides an easy-to-handle, visible reference that is especially valuable when I'm driving in heavy traffic.

Dianne Charron, RN, BSN

Pediatric care

A tip with teeth in it

As a school nurse, I see a lot of children who have loose baby teeth. Sometimes a tooth is so loose I have to pull it out so the child won't swallow it. To ease the child's fear and pain, I apply a small amount of benzocaine on the gum around the tooth. The benzocaine numbs the area so I can pull the tooth quickly and easily.

Tonya Rhodes, RN, BSN

Nursing reminder

A breast-feeding mother should alternate breasts each time she begins to breast-feed her baby. To help her remember which breast to use for the start of her baby's next feeding, suggest she put a small safety pin on the cup of her bra. After each feeding, she should move the pin to the other side to remind her to start with the other breast next time.

Bonnie Handerhan, RN, BSN

6 ASSESSMENT

Obtaining a history

Nursing history helper

To help you remember all the pertinent information you need to take a complete, systematic nursing history, use a pocket-sized card as a guide. Here's how to make one:

First, list the categories you wish to include. For example:

- Vital statistics
- Patient's understanding of illness
- Indication of expectations
- Social and cultural history
- Significant data.

Then type these subjects, with questions or specific items to ask the patient about, on both sides of a 5" x 7" card. Take the card to your hospital's print shop or a local printer and have it reduced in size (to about 3" x 5") and laminated to withstand the wear and tear of daily use.

The card is handy, easy to use, and lasts for years.

F. Kate Davis, RN

Quick assessment

When you need to make a patient assessment in a hurry and still obtain a maximum amount of information, try the 3-step SPADE technique.

First, determine the patient's status (or progress) in relation to his admitting diagnosis.

Next, assess his general status with SPADE:

Sleep
Pain
Activity
Diet
Elimination.

Finally, determine his most important request for assistance: "What's the most important thing you'd like to have help with today?"

This abbreviated assessment will help you in reviewing medical orders with doctors and in planning and implementing nursing care.

E. Jane Mezzanotte, RN, MSN

Medication board

Many of the patients we see in the emergency department don't know the names of medications they're taking. To help us get this information, we made a medication board. We glued samples of the most common pills and capsules on the board and labeled them. The patient can easily identify his medication, and we can record this information in his chart.

A word of caution: As soon as possible, double-check your information with the patient's doctor. And make sure the board is stored in a locked room or cabinet when it's not being used.

Maureen Dew, RN

Drug identification

Nurse: *"What drugs are you taking?"*
Patient: *"A little white pill."*

Sound familiar? Some suggestions from the clinical nurse coordinator of pediatric neurology at the Medical College of Georgia, Augusta, can help patients identify their medications.

One suggestion is to make a drug display board. Gather old copies of the *Physician's Desk Reference* (PDR) and cut out pictures of the drugs most frequently prescribed for your patients. If you're a neurology nurse, for example, you'd cut out pictures of Dilantin, Phenobarbital, and so on. Tape the pictures on a piece of cardboard and write the drug name beneath each.

If you don't have old copies of the PDR, ask the doctor to write a prescription for one pill of each medication your patients are likely to be taking. Place these pills inside the compartments of a fishing-lure box or a plastic box designed to hold nails and screws. Again, label each drug. (Be sure to store this container safely.)

Identifying liquid medications is more difficult. This suggestion may help: gather clear plastic bottles from the pharmacy and put 1 oz of the appropriate medication in each. Label the bottles and secure them side by side in a Styrofoam or balsawood base.

Once you have your drug display, show it to your patients and ask them to point to the drugs they're taking. Chances are they'll recognize their medications, or at least narrow the choice to a small group.

Diane G. Batts, RN

Performing physical examinations

Simon says

For a fun and easy way to assess pediatric trauma patients, play "Simon Says." Give your patient easy commands to follow, such as "Simon says, *'Say your name,'*" or "Simon says, *'Squeeze my hands.'*" Just for fun, throw in unnecessary commands, such as "Simon says, *'Say Pinocchio.'*" When I played this game with a 4-year-old who was involved in an automobile accident, she stopped crying and wanted to play the game over and over.

Renee Mills, RN

Isolated assessment

Being in isolation is no fun, especially for a child. To help me assess what he's thinking as well as how he's feeling, I do this:

Before entering the patient's room for the first time, I draw a nose and smile on my mask. Each time I enter the room thereafter, I ask him what I should draw. If he asks for a frown instead of a smile, I understand that all is not well and we talk about what's on his mind.

This gives me a chance to stem any fears or misconceptions before they become big problems. And my just being there wards off loneliness for a while.

Marie M. Shanahan, RN

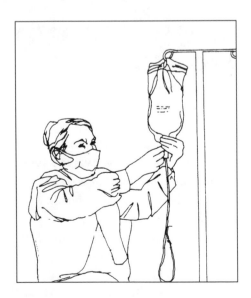

Picture story

Even careful documentation of a patient's skin condition doesn't always tell the story as clearly as possible. That's a good reason to include a "Rule of Nines" form—minus the numbers—with your written notes in your nursing care plan.

Indicate all skin abnormalities on the anatomical form by marking the appropriate areas with red ink. Also write a brief description of the abnormality, including size, appearance, type of wound, and so forth. This gives a picture that's truly worth a thousand words.

Pat Elswick, RN

Peripheral pulses: Hear the difference

You may have difficulty detecting arterial peripheral pulses with a Doppler ultrasound stethoscope. Try placing the probe at a 45-degree angle instead of at a 90-degree angle. The pulses will sound louder—sometimes twice as loud—because blood is flowing more directly toward the probe. That can make a big difference if the patient has peripheral vascular disease.

Debbie Metzler, RN, CCRN, MSN

Marking pulses

When using a Doppler ultrasound stethoscope, try marking the patient's peripheral pulses by applying white liquid correction fluid to the skin. The fluid won't dissolve, as ink does, with frequent applications of the gel used to obtain Doppler readings.

Linda Graves Allen, RN, BSN

X marks the pulse

Locating pedal and posttibial pulses can be time-consuming. After I find them, I use a felt-tip pen to mark an X over a palpable pulse and a D over a pulse that's detectable by a Doppler ultrasound stethoscope only. This not only helps the nurse on the next shift, but it also allows us to determine quickly if the pulse has worsened or improved.

Christine Ozoro, RN, BSN

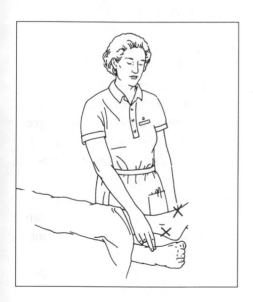

Time check

To assess a patient's capillary refill time, press down on his nail bed, release, then say the words "capillary refill." By the time you've said

that, normal color should have returned to his nail.

Patti Shewbart-Llewellyn, RN

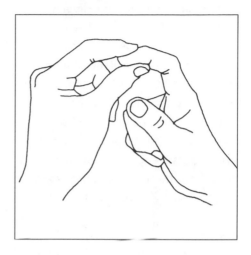

Cushion the noise

If you ever have to take a patient's blood pressure in an ambulance, air-ambulance plane, or some other noisy place, remember this tip: Put a pillow under the patient's antecubital area first. The pillow seems to cut out the distracting noise and allows you to get an accurate blood pressure reading.

Stephen M. Keller, EMT

Lung assessment

I've found a good way to demonstrate the sound of rales to new staff nurses. I pour a carbonated soft drink into a paper cup and tell the nurses to listen to the soft drink while it fizzes. They'll hear a good imitation of rales.

Joe Niemczura, RN, MS

Telltale tape

Once you've inserted an endotracheal tube, it's difficult to tell if it's staying in place or if it's slipping out of position. To see at a glance whether or not the tube has moved, put a small piece of adhesive tape around the tube so that one end of the tape touches the patient's lip or naris. Then if the tube moves out of position, you'll know because it will have pulled the tape from the patient's lip or naris.

Jacqueline Zabresky, RN

Neuro kit

On our neurosurgical unit, we are frequently asked to gather items for assessing cranial nerve function, so we made up an assessment kit.

The kit is a plastic basket with a handle (similar to an I.V. tray) containing cotton, safety pins, pennies, keys, peppermint, reflex hammer, tuning fork, pencil, tongue blade, blocks, and an ophthalmoscope. For added convenience, we mark each item with the name of the cranial nerve function it tests. The easy-to-tote kit saves us time when a neurosurgical test is called for.

Barbara Martin, RN

Lighting up at work

I keep a small, disposable flashlight (the kind sold for key chains) attached to my stethoscope. I use it for neurologic checks and for looking in the patient's throat. The flashlight is also a good distraction for younger patients. It's inexpensive and comes in various colors.

Nancy Kunz, SN

Getting a reaction

Here's a way to check for pupil reactivity without a penlight. First, turn on all the lights in the room and have your patient look directly at you with both eyes. Then, cover one of his eyes with your hand, watching for dilation (accommodation) in the other eye. Then, remove your hand and watch for constriction (direct light reflex) in the eye you'd covered. You can test the other eye the same way.

Lisa Inman, BSN

Squeezing for strength

Here's a quick way to check the strength of a patient's handgrip: Roll up a blood pressure cuff, pump it up slightly, and have the patient squeeze it while measuring the millimeters of mercury. Do the same thing with his opposite hand. The reading for the dominant hand may be higher by 10 to 20 mm Hg. This technique can help detect the slightest neurologic change, saving the patient from potential problems.

Dorothy M. Kellogg, RN

Hear here

If you suspect a patient has a fractured femur, hip, or pelvis, here's a way to confirm or refute your suspicions immediately:

Place your stethoscope on the patient's symphysis pubis and percuss each patella with your finger or a pen. On the side of the fracture, you'll hear a sound lower in volume and pitch than you'll hear on the unaffected side. (The reason is simple: The break in the bone interferes with the conduction of sound and decreases its frequency.)

Likewise, you can detect a fractured humerus, clavicle, or scapula by placing your stethoscope on the patient's sternum and percussing both funny bones (that is, the backs of the elbows where the ulnar nerve rests against a prominence of the humerus).

This technique is especially helpful for nurses who work in nursing homes or on geriatric units and need to assess a patient immediately after a fall.

Dash Pisarik Ziegler, RN, BSN

Exemplary exam

Before examining a patient's breasts, I warm a bottle of skin lotion in a basin of warm water. I apply some of the lotion to my hands. The lotion warms and softens my hands, which helps take the chill and friction out of the examination.

Kathleen Kerrigan, RN, BSN

Breast exam: Clear view

We've discovered an effective approach to teaching women how to do breast self-examinations. In each private examining room at our center, a mirror has been installed on the ceiling above the examination table. By watching in the mirror as we examine her breasts, the patient can see how it's done.

Sandee L. Kolodny, RN
Susan B. Fader, RN
Susan M. Poehlman, RN

Referral chart for pain control

You probably already use a standard pain-rating scale on the unit, but it may not be suitable for every patient. So you should ask the patient what scale he wants to use, then post it at his bedside. This will remind him and the nurses how to report his pain. And by posting the scale, you'll eliminate confusion; when a nurse sees the patient's scale, she'll immediately know what the rating he's given means to him.

Margo McCaffery, RN, MS, FAAN

Postpartum pointers

To assess a postpartum patient who's had a vaginal delivery, remember this: **F**or **E**very **L**ady **B**e **V**igilant. It will remind you to check her:
Fundus
Episiotomy site
Lochia
Breasts
Voiding.

Donald M. Grubb, RN, MSN, ARNP

Skin breakdown: Mirror image

When you're caring for a patient who can't turn over—such as a patient who's in traction—use a small mirror to check his heels for skin breakdown. Just lift his leg slightly, place the mirror under his heel, then assess the image.

Melissa A. White, RN, BSN

Keeping a stethoscope sterile

Preventing cross-contamination on the burn unit where I work is very important. So before I auscultate a patient's chest and abdomen, I place a rubber glove over my stethoscope's diaphragm. I can still hear heart, lung, and bowel sounds, as well as his pulse when I take a blood pressure reading—yet the diaphragm won't be contaminated with body fluids draining from a patient's wounds. When I'm finished, I dispose of the glove and wipe the diaphragm with an alcohol pad to help prevent cross-contamination.

Elizabeth A. Hendrix, RN, BSN

Obtaining accurate measure

A spill-proof cup

Do you have a patient who's unable to drink from a cup without spilling? Then this tip is just for him:

Punch a hole in the top of a sterile specimen cup, fill the cup with fluid, and put a straw through the hole. To disguise the cup, insert it into a regular paper cup and secure it with tape.

The cup's screw-on lid will prevent spills. And the measurement markings on the side of the cup will allow you to accurately assess the patient's intake.

Judi Williams, RN, BSN

In large measure

Tape measures sometimes aren't long enough to measure large abdomens, so use twill tape instead. Wrap the twill tape around the patient's abdomen, mark the tape with a pen or pencil, then measure it against the patient's own tape measure. After determining the patient's girth, throw the twill tape away to prevent cross-contamination.

Marie Fait, LPN

Eliminating guesswork

When you phone a doctor to report a patient's bleeding, do you have trouble describing how much? Many nurses do. Estimating isn't easy. Terms such as "bleeding heavily" could mean anywhere from 10 ml/hour to 5 or 10 times that much.

To avoid this problem, use a visual aid. Take three perineal pads. Onto the first, place 10 ml of blood from a syringe; onto the second, 30 ml; and onto the third, 60 ml. Then lay the three pads side by side, with cards underneath telling the amounts. Take a color photograph. Enlarge it to 8" x 10" and place copies on each unit as a ready reference.

Helen Gracey, RN
Michael Bruser, MD

A counterpoint

As you know, a patient with arterial peripheral vascular disease usually experiences leg pain that intensifies with walking. What you don't know is exactly how far the patient can walk without such pain. Vague descriptions such as "only a short distance," "not too far," or "from my house to the street corner" don't allow you to judge the severity of his disease.

For a more accurate assessment, have him count the number of steps he takes before he feels pain. This gives you objective data that you can use to measure the patient's progress.

Barbara Engram, RN, MSN

Picture this

A quick and easy way to measure intake is with a picture chart. Use a paper tray (such as those used to serve meals to patients in isolation) as the background. Cut in half the various sizes of paper or plastic cups, bowls, cartons, and so forth, and glue them to the tray. Then print the amount of fluids each holds underneath—for example, a carton of milk is 240 ml. Keep this chart on display at the nurses' station. This aid helps you measure intake at a glance when you pick up trays after meals.

Sarah Pettus, BSN

Writing on the wall

During postoperative orientation, we tell patients, family, and friends not to empty urinals and bedpans because we need to assess and measure the output. We also post a written reminder on the bathroom wall.

Rob Boyte, CNA

More than hems

A 6" hem gauge does more than just measure hems; it also helps measure the size of lacerations or contusions and the amount of bleeding or drainage on surgical dressings and casts.

Carry the gauge with you throughout the day—it takes up no more room in your pocket than a pen or bandage scissors.

Diane Klaiber, RN

Oximeter probe: Signal problems

An oximeter probe's signals may take several minutes to register on a baby with chubby feet. Here's a way to solve the problem:

Briskly rub the baby's foot with your hands or apply a warm, wet washcloth for a few minutes. Then attach the oximeter probe. The increased circulation and temperature help the probe work more effectively. And if you place a sock over the probe, the signals will stay on line.

Terrilynn Quillen, RN

In good measure

Unused nitroglycerin paste measuring papers come in handy when measuring the size of small wounds or lesions. Calibrated in ½" increments, the papers are plentiful on most cardiac units.

Karen L. Harris, RN

Accurate measurement

When I have a surgical patient with a Jackson-Pratt drain, I use a 60-ml, catheter-tipped syringe to aspirate the contents of the drain. That way, I get accurate input and output measurements, plus the fluid is self-contained.

Patricia Striggles, RN, BSN

Pupil paper

Determining a patient's pupil size is an important part of neurologic checks. But in recording the size, terminology may not be specific. For instance, a pupil that appears "moderate" in size to one person, may appear "dilated" to someone else.

To estimate and record pupil size more accurately, make a chart of pupil sizes on electrocardiogram paper. A pinpoint pupil is 1 mm—the size of one small square. A moderately sized pupil is 5 mm—the size of a large square. A fully dilated pupil is 8 or 9 mm. Keep the pupil-size chart at the nurses' station for quick reference.

Frances Marshall, RN

Get it straight

When you need to measure urine output with a urine meter, be sure to get it straight—the urine meter, that is. If the meter is tilted, the urine in the meter could overflow into the collection bag, making the measurement inaccurate. So take a moment to be sure the meter is hanging straight. It will save minutes later.

T. Jesaitis, SN

Bedpan lining

When careful stool measurements are ordered for a patient with gross rectal bleeding, try collecting specimens this way. First, rinse a bedpan with water. Next, press a large plastic bag into the contours of the pan, so the bag's edges form a collar over the edge of the pan. (The moisture in the pan keeps the bag in place.)

After the patient has passed the stool, lift the bag out of the pan and place it in the measuring container. Neither blood nor stool clings to either the bedpan or the container. This increases accuracy while eliminating cleanup.

To reduce odor, twist and tie the bag. You can save the specimen in a tied bag without telltale odors or much change in color.

Ruth P. Whitney, RN

Ideas that stick

Another type of sticker makes it easy for you to keep track of the amount of drainage in your patient's Hemovac. The sticker, which you place on top of the vacuum unit, should have room to record the patient's output for each shift over several days. It could look like this:

Output sticker

Date:	Date:
7-3:	7-3:
3-11:	3-11:
11-7:	11-7:
Date:	Date:
7-3:	7-3:
3-11:	3-11:
11-7:	11-7:

You record the amount of drainage on the appropriate line whenever you empty the container. Anyone who wants to know the patient's total drainage output can simply look at the sticker rather than having to search through the patient's chart.

Elizabeth Ward, RN

Penrose drainage

To collect wound drainage from a Penrose drain, place an ostomy appliance over the drain, taking care not to irritate the suture line. The drainage will accumulate in the appliance away from the patient's skin. This not only prevents skin breakdown and decreases dressing changes, but it also allows you to evaluate the color, consistency, and amount of drainage in the appliance.

Lana Sue Zinkon, RN

Tracking lab results with ease

We've devised a chart that makes noticing and evaluating changes in laboratory results easier, especially when patients need frequent blood tests. On a sheet of paper, we write the name of the test and the range of normal values. Then we draw several columns on the right, labeling each at the top with the date and time of testing. We record the values in those columns, so we can quickly spot trends and abnormal results.

Lourie Moore, RN, BSN

Check the chart

Do you ever find that another nurse describes a wound drainage as moderate, when you'd consider it small? Or do you have trouble visualizing the size of an inflamed area that someone else describes as 4 cm?

One way to take the guesswork out of such situations is to have everyone use a standard chart for reference. The chart used in labor and delivery to measure cervical dilation is ideal. Simply display the chart where it's accessible to the entire unit staff and have them refer to the chart for assessment of wound drainage or measurement of any area up to 10 cm in size.

The use of such a chart makes charting simpler and more consistent, saving time in shift reports.

Mary S. Hall, RN

Collections on the move

If you're transporting a patient who has a nasogastric tube and you need to collect drainage from the tube while you're moving him, try this: Secure a disposable plastic glove to the end of the tube with a rubber band or piece of tape. The glove will collect the drainage, and later, you can easily empty the drainage from the glove into a cup for measuring.

Kimberly A. Stotts, RN, BSN

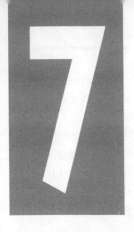

PROCEDURES

Sore mouth: Cosmetic solution

I had a patient with an endotracheal tube who developed pressure ulcers at the corners of her mouth from the twill tie that secured the tube. I solved this problem by placing cosmetic makeup wedges under the twill tie, with the wide sides closest to her mouth. The inexpensive

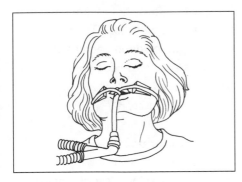

wedges kept the tie from touching the patient's skin and distributed the tie's pressure more evenly. Of course, I changed the wedges daily or if they became soiled. (They're washable in soap and water, and they dry quickly.)

Tom Baker, RN, CRTT, BSN

Dental device for oral suctioning

We had a patient in our unit with multiple sclerosis who could move only his eyelids, lips, and tongue. Because he had trouble clearing oral secretions, he needed to be suctioned every 10 minutes. His inability to clear secretions was a frightening experience for him, and the frequent suctioning was time-consuming for us.

So we obtained a suction tip from our dental clinic, adapted it to our wall suction tubing, set the suction on an intermittent low level, then placed the tip in the patient's mouth. (The tip doesn't create enough suction to pull lips or oral mucosa into the device.) This way,

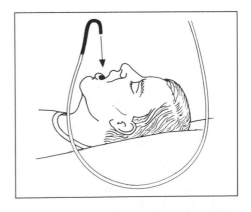

he could direct the secretions to the tube himself, decreasing his anxiety—and saving us time.

Thomas J. Wenzel, RN, BSN

No-mess mouth care

Giving mouth care to a patient who must lie flat in bed isn't easy—especially the rinsing and spitting. But here's a way to avoid the mess:

After the patient's teeth are brushed, offer him mouthwash or water through a straw. Then have him use the same straw to expel the mouthwash or water into an emesis basin.

Although using a straw may be a bit awkward at first, patients usually master it quickly and become proficient in the ins *and* outs of rinsing and spitting with straws.

Kathy Scheeve, SN

Foam in the mouth

To remove blood from a patient's mouth, try a solution of half peroxide and half ginger ale. Just dip a toothbrush, mouth swab, or gauze into the solution, brush or wipe the

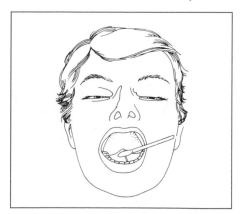

patient's mouth, and let the blood foam away. Follow with a plain water rinse.

This method works especially well on unconscious patients. And most conscious patients find it a pleasant mouth rinse.

Janice Heistand, RN, CCRN

Using dental floss

If your patient has trouble using dental floss to perform his own oral hygiene, you can help him this way.

Tie one end of some floss to the end of a tongue blade and the other end of the floss to the end of *another* tongue blade. (Or make pinholes through the ends of two tongue blades; then thread one end of the floss through one pinhole and the other end of the floss through the other pinhole. Knot the ends of the floss to prevent them from slipping through the pinholes.) Then hold one tongue blade in each hand, pull the floss taut, and floss your patient's teeth.

Marie A. Frasca, RN

Natural cleanser

Many times we clean a patient's mouth by swabbing it with papaya juice, a sponge, and a Toothette. Papaya juice, available at most health food stores, is a natural enzyme that removes most debris without injuring the patient's mouth. And no harm is done if the patient swallows some of the mouth "cleanser."

Afterward, we irrigate the patient's mouth with water.

Mary T. Knapp, RN

What a difference a tray makes

Reuse disposable dressing trays as oral hygiene trays; they have three compartments to store all the equipment you need to give patients good mouth care.

In one compartment, put 2" x 2" pieces of gauze; in another, pour your oral cleansing solution; and in the last compartment, store cotton swabs, tongue blades, petroleum jelly, and plastic Kelly forceps. (These forceps are small enough to reach into tiny areas and strong enough to grip the gauze firmly while you're cleaning the patient's mouth.)

The trays help keep supplies together, making mouth care much easier and neater.

Debbie Niemi, RN

Hiccup tip

Here's a sure cure for patients' hiccups. Take a cotton swab and gently massage the roof of the mouth, just beyond the spot where the soft and hard palates meet.

Phyllis Novitskie, RN, BSN

Keeping dentures in one piece

Before you brush or rinse a patient's dentures, put a towel in the sink. That way, the dentures won't break if you drop them.

Kay B. Stewart, RN, CS, MSN

Providing eye and ear care

Eye-opener

Need to improvise an eyecup if one isn't readily available? Use a sterile spoon—either teaspoon or tablespoon size. Fill the spoon with the eyewash solution. As the patient bends his head forward, place the spoon over the eye with the point resting on the inner corner of the eye. Then tell the patient to tip his head backward, open his eyelid, and wash the eye.

Your patient can use this improvisation at home or even away, as on a camping trip, for example.

La Donna Kolman, RN

An eye piece

Problem: A patient comes to the emergency department complaining of eye pain and photophobia. He won't let you put an eye patch on him because he's afraid it will put pressure on his eye.

Solution: Cut the bottom from a clean plastic cup, tape the rough edges, place the cup over the eye, and secure it with a piece of tape.

The cup protects the eye without actually touching it.

Sydney Anne Gambill, RN

Icy fingers

When the weight of a regular ice pack on the eyelid is too painful for a patient, make an "icy finger" ice pack instead.

Fill finger cots with water, tie them shut, and freeze them. Place two ice-filled cots inside a piece of 2" stockinette and pin or tape two pieces of twill tape to the stockinette—one at each end. Place the stockinette over the patient's eye and tie the twill tape at the top of the patient's head.

This icy finger pack is lighter than regular ice packs and stays in place itself so the patient can freely use both hands. We keep a supply of them in the freezer for fast and easy replacement.

Barbara Simonds, RN

Eyewash

Patients with eye traumas need copious eye irrigations. An easy and efficient way to give them is to attach I.V. tubing (without the needle) to 1 liter of normal saline solution, then use the tubing to direct the saline solution into the patient's eye. If necessary, you can regulate the stream by using the flow clamp.

Barbara Sosaya, RN, BSN

Lens lifter

Ever have to remove contact lenses from multiple trauma patients? The quickest and most painless way to do this is to use the suction tip of a glass eyedropper. By depressing the suction tip and gently applying it directly over the lens, you can lift the lens off the cornea quite easily.

Marleen Kaechele, RN

Safekeeping for contacts

Here's what I do when a patient who wears contact lenses forgets to bring his lens storage case to the hospital. I label two plastic medicine cups with the patient's name—marking one right and the other left—and fill each with about 5 ml of normal saline solution. I have the patient put his lenses into the appropriate cups. Then I secure gauze over each with a rubber band and put the cups in the patient's bedside cabinet. Later, I give the lenses to a family member so they can be properly stored at home.

Elizabeth Colello, RN, BSN

When seconds count

When suctioning an artificial airway, you shouldn't apply suction for longer than 15 seconds at a time.

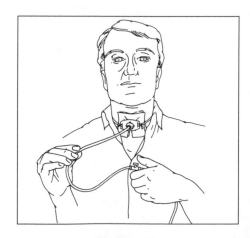

But how do you know when the seconds have passed? Use this technique from cardiopulmonary resuscitation (CPR).

During CPR, you count—"one, one thousand; two, one thousand; three, one thousand"—to mark off the seconds. Similarly, in suctioning, you can count, "one, one thousand; two, one thousand" and so on until the seconds have elapsed. Then remove the suction catheter.

Robert Hutson, RRT, EdD

Wrap, tape, and irrigate
To absorb leakage and keep the patient's shirt dry while you're irrigating his ear, try this: Wrap the long edge of a disposable diaper around the patient's neck—absorbent side up—and fasten it with the tape tab. Curve up the outer edge to catch any solution the diaper doesn't absorb.

You can use whatever size diaper fits your patient's neck.

Jackie Pederson, RN

Ear's relief
An oxygen cannula may cause skin breakdown on top of a patient's ear. If so, clear the area and cut a sterile bandage lengthwise. Place the bandage over the ear and rest the cannula on the gauze portion. That should relieve the pressure.

Cheryl Reich, RN

Caring for equipment

A suction tip
If you use a tonsil suction tip for mouth care, here's how to keep it clean between uses: Tape the cover of a 60-ml syringe to the back of the headboard. Then, after using the suction tip, place it in the syringe cover to keep it from falling onto the patient's bed or the floor.

When you change the tonsil suction tip, change the syringe cover, too.

Paula Chelewski, RN

Expired time
When I check inventory on the crash cart, I write each medication's expiration date on the inventory flow sheet. That way, expired medications are quickly noticed and discarded before they're used during a code.

Patty Swetnam, RN

Cleaning with cola
When a feeding tube becomes clogged with formula, unclog it with diet cola. Get a doctor's order first;

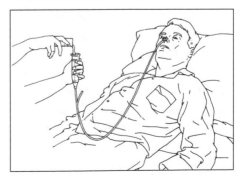

then flush the feeding tube with
1 oz of cola. Clamp the tube for
15 minutes. The cola will dissolve
the formula and unclog the tube.

Nina S. Ehle, RN

A feeding tube flush

Small-diameter enteral feeding tubes
often get clogged from the feeding
formula residue. To prevent this
residue buildup, we flush the tubes
every 4 hours (and each time the
feeding is interrupted or discontinued) with ⅝ oz of cranberry juice,
followed by ⅜ oz of water.

The acidic cranberry juice breaks
up the formula's residue, and the
water rinses away the juice, preventing sugar from crystallizing in the
tube.

Dee Adinaro, RN, MSN

Deodorizing drops

Want to eliminate odors from your
patients' urinals, bedpans, com-
modes, and suction bottles? Just
pour a few drops of mouthwash in
them. The unpleasant smells will disappear.

Janet D. Stolarz, LPN

Stop MAST contamination

Blood-soiled medical antishock
trousers (MAST) must be carefully
washed to prevent blood-transmit-
ted diseases. The *MAST Manual* sug-
gests using a washing machine with
medium-temperature water and
household detergents. It also sug-
gests closing the inflation/deflation
valves before washing.

But what if a valve's left open, or
opens inadvertently during the wash
cycle? The contaminated wash
water enters the chambers and is
difficult to remove.

To prevent this problem, follow
the procedure used at Community
Hospital of San Gabriel, Calif.: Place
a rubber stopper from the top of a
standard red-top Vacutainer in each
valve. The stopper seals the valve so
water can't enter the chambers.

Annals of Emergency Medicine,
June 1984

Preparing hot/cold therapy

Numbing a port site

A patient with an implanted port
may have some pain when you
insert a needle into the port. So I
briefly put ice chips over the port
site to numb the area. Then the
patient feels less discomfort.

Mitzi A. Llamas, RN

Cool pad

Here's a method of applying ice to a
patient's perineum after an episioto-
my:

First, cut a sanitary pad in half—
the short way—and soak the halves
in water until saturated. Then take
each half and fashion it into a 1"-
diameter roll. Next, cover the roll
with a 5" x 5" square of plastic

kitchen wrap and put it into the freezer.

When the roll is frozen, place one or two Tucks pads on the patient's perineum, put the frozen roll over the Tucks pads, and hold both roll and pad(s) in place with another whole sanitary pad.

Denise Houle, RN

Pillowcase treatments

If your patient needs to keep a heating pad or ice pack on the back of his neck or shoulder while he's lying in bed, just slip it inside his pillowcase—on top of the pillow.

Mary Kraft, RN, BSN

Warming hot packs

Use a slow-cooker to heat hot packs. Set it to the desired temperature, and you'll have moist hot packs readily available.

Joanne E. Gerson, RN

Refreezable cold packs

Fill plastic freezer bags half full with water, remove excess air, and freeze them. They're inexpensive, stay cold longer than the chemical packs, and are available in a variety of sizes for convenience.

Marguerite Quinn, RN

Packed for travel

After I had an excisional biopsy on my left breast, the doctor told me to apply an ice pack to the site.

Because I didn't want to stay in bed while the ice was applied, I made a "traveling ice pack."

I got two disposable rubber gloves, filled one with tepid water, and filled the other with ice and water. I tied both gloves shut with a long piece of gauze—one glove at each end of the gauze. Then I placed the ice-filled glove next to the biopsy site and let the other glove hang down my back. The two gloves counterbalanced each other so I could move about freely and still keep the ice pack in place.

Nancy Deveney, RN

Ice sealing

To improvise an ice pack, try using the kitchen appliance that seals a meal into a plastic bag. Fill a large-size bag with ice and seal it. Apply this pack to the affected area. The ice will melt, but the pack remains cool, with no leakage.

Place the bag of water in the freezer and you have an ice pack ready for the next injury. You can make a few in various sizes and keep them in the freezer at the hospital for your patients.

Sherri Sener, RN, BSN

Shoe covers: Frozen function

In our postanesthesia care unit, we often have patients who need ice applied to the operative site. We put ice packs in small plastic bags and then place them in operating room shoe covers. Shoe covers aren't as bulky as towels and the elastic keeps the bags tightly secured.

Tanja Singletary, RN

O₂ and jaws, too

In our recovery room, we use face tents to administer oxygen. We've found they can also be used to hold ice packs on the jaw or face of patients who've had surgery at these sites.

Lori Giverson, RN

Positioning patients

Fan-tastic idea

Here's a simple way to pull up a patient in bed. I fold a sheet lengthwise and place it on top of the fitted bottom sheet, starting at the head of the bed. Then I fanfold the excess at the foot of the bed. That way, one nurse can easily move a patient who's slipped down in the bed without running out of sheet.

Carrie Brown, RN

Pillow prop

When you're positioning a patient on his side in bed and you prop a pillow behind his back, does the pillow slip away? If so, untuck the drawsheet and place the pillow *under* the drawsheet. Then tuck the sheet back under the mattress. The pillow won't slip, and the patient will stay on his side.

Betty Ann Ulmer, RN

Comfortable position for eating

Because a cardiac catheterization patient has to lie flat and keep his leg straight and still, he may have difficulty eating. To solve the problem, I place his bed in reverse Trendelenburg's position so the patient can see his meal and eat it more comfortably. Some of my patients have even successfully eaten soup this way.

Thomas Hackett, RN, CCRN

Straight with a sheet

When a patient returns from an angiogram, he often needs to keep his leg straight for at least 8 hours. So I fold a sheet lengthwise and place it over the knee of the affected leg, then tuck the ends of the sheet under the mattress. This mild restraint helps the patient keep his leg straight without compromising skin integrity.

Nancy R. Redner, RN

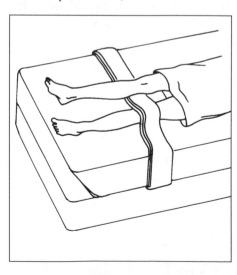

Cardiac catheterization: Staying straight

When I had trouble keeping my leg straight following cardiac catheterization, my daughter put a 14" strip of tape lengthwise over my knee. The tape was a lightweight restraint that served as an instant reminder whenever I started to bend my knee. (Of course, you wouldn't use tape on a patient with unhealthy skin.)

Janet R. Gerow, RN

Easy immobilizer

I use a full-length leg immobilizer to prevent hip flexion when a patient has an intra-aortic balloon catheter or an arterial line catheter in his femoral artery. Of course, I pad any potential pressure areas and check the patient's pulses every hour.

Judy Gilmore, RN

Leg lift

When I'm in a hurry to prep a patient's leg for surgery, I attach a gynecologic stirrup to the operating room bed and place the patient's foot in it. This also allows me to reposition the bed, if I need to, without disturbing the prepped leg. Another benefit: When I'm ready to remove the stirrup after draping, I can do so with one hand, holding the prepped leg with the other.

Mary Valley, RN, CNOR

Weigh to go

On the intensive care unit where I work, most of our patients have orders for daily weights and complete bed rest. To save us time and effort and to spare the patient unnecessary movement, we always try to be prepared for daily weights ahead of time.

For example, when we hear a new patient is being admitted, or when a patient is temporarily in another area of the hospital, we place a bed scale sling on the bed. When the patient arrives or returns, we're ready to obtain an accurate weight.

Mary Boris, RN

Making occupied beds

A sheet feat

Changing the drawsheet on the bed of an immobilized patient is not only a difficult task for you, it's an uncomfortable experience for your patient as well.

To make the procedure a little easier on everyone, do it this way: Untuck the old drawsheet and attach one side edge of the new drawsheet to one side edge of the old one with three safety pins. If possible, have the patient lift himself with an over-bed trapeze. Then pull the old drawsheet across the bed. The new drawsheet will follow and replace the old one—wrinkle-free—underneath the patient. Just remove the pins, tuck in the new drawsheet, and you're finished.

Pat Wheeler, RN

Two tasks at once

When I use a bed scale to weigh a patient, I place new linen on his bed while he's still suspended on the scale's sling. Changing the linen when I weigh him not only saves time, but also prevents the patient from being disturbed more than necessary.

Patty Swetnam, RN

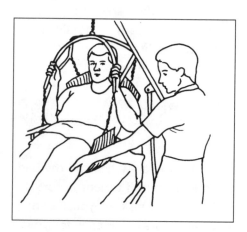

Padded pull sheet

When you're making the bed of a bedridden patient who needs a disposable underpad, prepare his bed as you normally would—with one exception. Instead of placing the pad on top of the drawsheet directly under the patient, sandwich it between the drawsheet layers.

This technique will mean fewer soiled bottom sheets, thereby saving you time and cutting your hospital's linen consumption. It will also add to your patient's comfort, because paper from the pad won't cling to his skin.

Janet Markey, RN

On a roll

Changing a bed with the patient in it means a lot of tugging, rolling, confusion, and—for some patients—pain. But you can save yourself and your patient some trouble and discomfort by partially *premaking* his bed on an empty bed, if one's available.

Layer the bed linens (including disposable underpads, lift sheets, and drawsheets) on the empty bed just as if you were going to make it—but don't tuck the linen in. Starting at one side, roll the linen into a tube. Place the linen tube alongside the patient's bed. Then, roll the patient to the far side of the bed, push the dirty linen toward the patient, and roll the new linen tube out onto his bed. All the layers of new linens will be in place on one side of the bed, and you can tuck them in. Roll the patient back and finish pulling off the old linen and tucking in the new linen.

If your patient is in balance-suspension traction, you may find it easier to roll the linen from the top of the bed to the bottom instead of from side to side.

Gail Chark, RN

Managing elimination and drainage

Avoiding tube twist

In the busy urology-surgical unit where I work, we use clear, plastic drinking straws to prevent small-bore drainage tubing from twisting and kinking. Here's how: We cut the straw to the length of the tubing, make a slit down the length of the straw, and wrap the straw around the tubing. Then we secure the straw with the clear plastic tape so that the staff can view the tube and the drainage. The straw decreases time spent cleaning the patient and fixing the tubing, and improves patient comfort.

John R. Kincade, RN

Unconventional urinal

When I take a male patient who uses a wheelchair for a walk, I bring a baby bottle so that he can use it as a urinal, if necessary. The patient appreciates my thoughtfulness and the bottle works great—it's small, leakproof, easy to clean, and discreet.

Vicki Patterson, LVN

Fitting connections

When connecting plastic tubing of uneven sizes, such as a drain to a collection system, use an indwelling urinary catheter. Because it has a graduated diameter and is flexible, an indwelling urinary catheter can be cut to any length. What's more, you can use sterile technique when connecting the tubing because indwelling urinary catheters are packaged in sterile wrappers.

Carole Oberle, RN, CETN, MSN

Bedtime stroll

If your patient is bothered by having to urinate frequently during the night, help him walk about for at least 10 minutes, 1 to 2 hours before bedtime. This will markedly decrease his trips to the bathroom because muscular activity helps to mobilize fluid.

Casey Renz, RN, BS

Solution for emergency irrigation

In the emergency department where we work, we've devised an irrigation setup to help us lavage patients who have massive hemorrhaging from a gastrointestinal bleed. We connect a 1,000- or 3,000-ml bag of normal saline solution to I.V. tubing that fits the air lumen of a Salem sump tube. Then we irrigate and suction as needed. This frees us to do other tasks, such as drawing blood and starting I.V.s It's been a timesaving and lifesaving idea.

Debbie Tate, LPN
Judy Lance, RN

Lighter lavage

Try this tip for gastric lavage with a Salem sump tube. Set up a 1,000-ml bag of normal saline solution with I.V. tubing. Insert the tubing into the blue air port of the Salem sump tube. Next, connect the suction port of the Salem sump tube to continuous low suction, and open the saline line. Now you don't have to use a 60-ml catheter-tip syringe to withdraw the lavage solution— making the procedure more comfortable for the patient.

Marilyn Prout, RN

Easier catheterization

When you're catheterizing a male patient, try using a lubricant that comes in a sterile catheter-tipped syringe or tube. Gently squeeze the lubricant directly into the urethral canal. This will ensure that the lubricant is where it's needed, which will help you pass the tube through the canal.

Polly Zimmermann, RN, BSN

Apply condom catheter

Applying a condom catheter can be tricky—pubic hair can get caught in the adhesive tape, hurting the patient when the catheter is removed. So now I cut a 1" circle out of a disposable (paper) washcloth. Then I pull the patient's penis through the hole, making sure all his pubic hair remains under the washcloth. Finally, I apply the catheter and tear away the washcloth.

Margaret Blanchard, LPN

Adaptable external catheter for men

Some male patients are unable to use a condom catheter for urine collection. I've adapted a drainable fecal incontinence collector for this purpose.

Here's what to do: First, shave the patient's pubic area if necessary. Then open the appliance as directed and place the shaft of his penis through the opening. The wide portion of the skin barrier material should cover his pubic bone. Smooth out the skin as you press the barrier material against the scrotum. Cap the plastic pouch and attach it to a collection bag. Make sure you assess the patient for skin irritation, and change the appliance every 2 days.

Evelyn M. Dash, RN

No cath? No problem

When you have a male patient who's incontinent but can't use an indwelling urinary catheter, try a newborn-size disposable diaper instead.

Just gently wrap the diaper around the patient's entire penis, secure the tape tab, and fold over or tape the open end shut.

The disposable diapers are more

comfortable and safer than conventional incontinent pads and pins, and they look better under trousers than bulky rubber pants. Also, after the patient has voided, you can weigh the diaper for an accurate intake and output measurement. And before applying a fresh diaper, all you (or he) need do is clean the genital area.

Judith B. Schwandt, RN

Easy catheterization

If a female patient can't lie in the supine position for catheterization, try turning her on her side and bending her knees up toward her chest. You'll be able to see the urethral meatus easily, and the patient will be more comfortable during the procedure.

Katie Swett, RN, BSN

Cath care comfort

Here's a tip for catheterizing a female patient who has a fractured hip or who finds the dorsal recumbent position uncomfortable:

Turn the patient on her left side in the Sims' position, with the right knee and thigh drawn up, if possible. Place a sterile drape over her buttocks, covering the rectal area. Then separate the labia and proceed to catheterize her.

Elderly patients especially find this position more comfortable than the traditional position.

Sonja Feist, RN, MS

No more odor

If you notice a strong, unpleasant odor emanating from a urine drainage bag at a patient's bedside, try this: Add 10 ml of hydrogen peroxide to the bag every time you empty it. The hydrogen peroxide prevents bacteria from forming in the bag; hence, no odor. It also prevents bag discoloration and urine turbidity.

Jo Ann M. Camasso, RN, CNA, BSN

The sole answer

My patients include some women with spinal cord injuries who have indwelling urinary catheters. Changing the catheter is difficult because I have no one to help position the patient, so I can't get a clear view of her urethra. To solve this problem, I carry a pair of tennis or crepe-soled shoes with my equipment.

I position the patient on her back and put the shoes on her feet. I then place her feet close to her buttocks and let her legs open. The rubbery soles of the shoes keep her feet from slipping, and I can see what I'm doing. This makes catheterization quicker, and easier on the patient, too.

C. Bess Farrell, RN, BSN

Catheter correction

When you catheterize a female patient, have two catheters of the appropriate size with you. That way, if you mistakenly insert the first catheter into the vagina, you can leave it there as a guide while you insert the other one. This saves time and prevents making the same mistake twice.

Edwina A. McConnell, RN, PhD

A viewpoint on catheterization

One of the biggest problems in catheterizing a woman patient without assistance is getting a good view of her perineal area. So try placing a bedpan or fracture pan upside down on the bed with a pad over it. Then position the patient's buttocks on the pan. You'll be able to see the area more clearly, and catheter insertion will be easier.

Cathie Holtzinger, RN

In control again

Pass this hint to a patient who's having trouble voiding after his urinary catheter is removed: Tell him to blow bubbles through a straw into a glass half-filled with water. The water sounds should help the patient void easily again.

Florence Mackinnon, NA

Left holding the bag

Patients who are receiving continuous bladder irrigation sometimes have trouble ambulating with the drainage bag. If they have an I.V., they often hook the bag to a knob

on the pole. Then the bag is too high for proper drainage.

To solve this problem, we put a square piece of heavy cardboard over the legs at the base of the I.V. pole. This "floor" gives patients a place to rest the bag and still maintain proper drainage while they're ambulating. To secure the bag, attach its clip hook to the pole, and lightly wrap gauze or tape around the bag and pole.

Doug Burgay, CNB, SNI

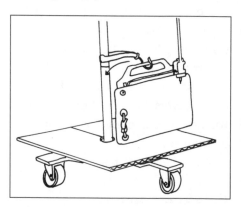

Pantastic idea

The next time a patient who's in a chair or wheelchair needs a bedpan, try reversing the position of the pan. The reversed pan supports the patient's thighs without digging into them, as it does in its regular position. Also, there's less chance of spillage with the pan in the reverse position.

Loretta A. Debus, RN

Urine-free cast

To prevent urine contamination of a hip-spica cast, cover its crotch area with a polyethylene drape. The drape's hypoallergenic adhesive sticks to the cast and won't irritate the patient's skin.

Ann Cunningham, RN

Tender-touch terry

Here are some ways to make a urinal more comfortable for a man:

To protect the patient's scrotum and penis from irritation, place a terry-cloth wristband on the opening of the urinal. And to prevent irritation of the patient's inner thighs, slip a terry-cloth headband around the middle of the urinal.

A money-saving hint: Rather than buying the bands, make them. Sew a 2" x 3" piece of stretch terry cloth together to make the wristband. And sew a 2" x 4" piece of terry cloth together to make the headband.

The bands can be easily removed for laundering whenever necessary.

Dale S. Lohmann, RN, MSN

No-friction fracture pan

Before giving a fracture pan to a patient, apply some body lotion to the pan rim. The lotion will decrease the friction—and the pain—of using the pan.

Deborah Wood, RN
Helen Kelsey, RN

Bedpan comfort

When you take a patient off a plastic bedpan, does his skin stick to the seat? If so, try sprinkling some powder on the rim of the bedpan before he uses it. And a light dusting of powder on a patient's legs before applying antiembolism stockings helps the stockings go on easier.

Nila C. E. Sadek, RN

Soft tube

If you're having trouble passing a Salem sump tube because it's too large for your patient's nares, try running *warm* water over the last 5" to 6" of the tube. The water softens the tube, minimizing trauma and discomfort to your patient. Also, water left clinging to the tube helps advance it.

Deborah Lamb Mechanick, RN

No overflow woes

When a fracture pan overflows, changing the bed linens can be painful for your patient. But you can easily prevent such overflow by siphoning urine away from the fracture pan. Here's how:

Get some straight tubing, a 30-ml syringe, and a urine collector. Place one end of the tubing into the fracture pan, the other end onto the syringe's needle. Position your patient on the pan and place the urine collector at a lower level.

As the patient starts to void, pull the syringe's plunger back. This will create suction and start a flow of urine. Remove the syringe from the tubing, and quickly place the tubing into the collector.

Besides reducing your patient's discomfort, this technique will reduce your hospital's linen usage. You can also use the technique when giving perineal care.

Linda Hooker, RN

Tissue, tissue, everywhere...

Do you dislike having toilet tissue sitting everywhere and anywhere in a patient's room? And no matter where it is, it's always out of reach when needed.

The solution? Have your maintenance department install toilet tissue holders on an arm of each bedside commode. Then the tissue will always be where it's needed. And even though it's still visible, the tissue's new location seems more appropriate than the windowsill, or the bedside stand, or the dresser top, or....

Sandra Holdt, RN

Clean dressing for pressure ulcer

When a patient has a sacral pressure ulcer, the bottom of his dressing is near his rectum and may become soiled, especially if the patient is incontinent. To avoid this, I place a sanitary napkin over the rec-

tal area to absorb feces. Frequent napkin changes keep the dressing clean.

Gail Dittes, RN

Bring on the bran

No one—neither patient nor nurse—enjoys a laxative or an enema. Yet, for long-term bedridden patients on a solid food diet, establishing bowel habits presents problems.

Here's a solution to some of those problems: unprocessed bran. With patients who are immobile for long periods and who have no dietary restrictions, sprinkle 1 to 2 teaspoons of bran on their food or in their fruit juice for each meal daily. Then leave the bran container at their bedside so they can regulate the amount to suit their own needs, perhaps decreasing it to twice daily. Patients using bran have no cramping, as they do after a laxative, and they don't have discomfort. And, oh, the nursing hours saved by the decreased need for enemas!

Myra B. Alexander, RN

Heat-a-fleet

Before giving a Fleet (or similar) enema, place the unit in a microwave oven on a low setting for about 20 seconds. This will warm the liquid and make the enema much easier to administer.

Jane M. Johnson, RN
E.J. Richey, NA

Enema aid

If a patient with a weak anal sphincter needs an enema, try using a
baby-bottle nipple to hold the
catheter of the enema tubing in
place. Enlarge the nipple's hole,
pointing it toward the patient's
anus. Then pass the catheter inside
the nipple and out through its hole.
The nipple will act as a shield and
will help the patient retain the
enema.

    Cathy A. Lawniczak, RN, BSN

Relaxing routine

Ever have difficulty inserting a rectal
tube for an enema when the
patient's apprehensive? First, explain
the procedure to the patient, then
place a warm, wet cloth against his
anal sphincter for a few minutes.
This helps the patient relax his
sphincter muscle, permitting easy
insertion of the well-lubricated
tube.

    Renee Berke, RN

Flexible idea

Giving enemas to patients in traction who can't turn from side to
side can be difficult. To solve this
problem, I place a rubber straight
catheter on the end of a Fleet
enema, clear the catheter of air,
then insert it. Extending the length
of the enema tube makes the procedure easier for the patient and
the nurse.

    Gladys M. Thorsell, RN

Collecting specimens

Collection without contamination

When I need a urine specimen from
a female patient, I ask her to clean
her perineal area with a washcloth
and soap and then use the packaged
wipe in the collection kit. This mini-
mizes the number of inaccurate cul-
ture readings.

    Wendi A. Arce, RN

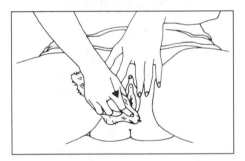

Tool for diabetic testing

When I'm teaching a diabetic
patient how to check his blood glucose level, I suggest that he keep a
small mirror with his other supplies.
Then, when he pricks his finger, he
can place the mirror under his fin-

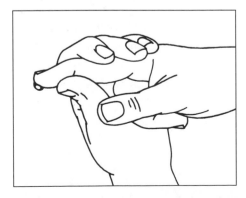

ger and see the blood without rotating his finger and possibly losing the blood.

Nanette I. Woodrum, RN

Warm-up in 30 seconds

Before you stick a patient's finger for a blood glucose test, wrap the finger in a warm, damp washcloth for 30 seconds. This will increase circulation to the area and will reduce the chance of having to stick him more than once.

Jamie Schoonover, RN, BSN

Pick up the tab

I found an easy way to pick up glucose-monitoring test strips. Just fold ½" of the strip opposite the test pad. Now you have a small tab that's easy to grasp and use. This also will decrease the chance of flipping the strip over, contaminating the pad, and having to repeat the test.

Pamela Miller, LPN

Pinchless tourniquet

To avoid pinching a patient's skin when you tie a rubber tourniquet around his upper arm, tie it over the sleeve of his gown. The sleeve acts as a buffer, allowing you to tie the tourniquet without pinching the skin.

Nancy J. Davidson, RN

Go with the flow

Next time you're taking a blood sample from a patient and the flow stops, loosen the tourniquet momentarily. If the tourniquet is too tight, it may impede arterial blood flow. Releasing pressure this way usually starts the blood flowing again.

Bertha L. Clarke, RN, CEN, BSN

Fast access to Vacutainers

Because we draw our own blood specimens in the emergency department, we keep all the necessary equipment on a phlebotomy tray. But we used to misplace our Vacutainers. Here's how we solved the problem:

We taped several tongue blades onto the tray's center handle, leaving about 4" of each blade sticking up from the top of the handle. The tongue blades hold the Vacutainers. So now we don't have to waste time looking for them—they're quickly and easily accessible.

Polly Zimmermann, RN, BSN

One stick is enough

Here's a way to draw blood for arterial blood gases (ABGs) and other blood work with one puncture and one needle:

Insert an ABG syringe with a rubber syringe-tipped cap into the Vacutainer sleeve. Puncture the top cap with the interior spike of the Vacutainer needle, and leave the syringe in place. Perform the arterial puncture using the Vacutainer sleeve and needle as if it were an ABG syringe.

When you've collected enough blood, exchange the syringe for the Vacutainer tubes. The rubber spike protector inside the Vacutainer will prevent blood flow during the exchange.

Paul J. Mathews, RRT, EdS, FCCM

One stick will do

Many patients who arrive in our emergency department in critical condition have limited sites for laboratory blood draws. So I attach a stopcock to a 1 ½" needle and connect the arterial blood gas (ABG) syringe to the vertical port of the stopcock. Then I insert the needle into the artery. After drawing the blood for ABGs, I turn off the stopcock and carefully disconnect the syringe. Then I attach a syringe to draw blood for other laboratory values. This way, I only have to stick the patient once to get all the blood I need.

Yvonne D. Sabyan, RN

No *draw*backs

When drawing blood from a patient with delicate veins, I use a 23-gauge winged-tip needle instead of a regular Vacutainer needle. The winged-tip needle is steadier and helps prevent damage to veins.

Lt. Roy Fukuoka, BSN

No more needle sticks

One of our nurses recently sustained a needle stick when drawing blood from a hemodialysis access port. To prevent this from happening again, we now put a 3-way stopcock between the access port and the hemodialysis tubing. This way we can draw blood without accidental needle sticks.

Jan Barnes, RN, CHN, BSN

Easy sample

After unsuccessfully trying to obtain a midstream urine sample from an elderly patient, we came up with an unorthodox solution. We had the patient sit on a commode chair. Then we put the chair's collection container on the floor under the seat. This gave us plenty of room to clean her perineum and collect the sample.

Maryanne Kehoe, RN
Bill Cramer, RN

Geriatricks

Collecting a urine specimen from an elderly woman patient when you can't get an order for an indwelling or straight catheter can be difficult. So try using a pediatric urine bag. Tape the bag over the patient's perineum. It holds about 50 to 60 ml of urine—sufficient for most tests.

Debora J. Burke, RN

Collection glove

Here's how we can collect urine specimens from incontinent male patients in the geriatric facility where I work: We turn an examining glove inside out and place it over the patient's penis. After taping the glove in place, we put a disposable adult incontinence pad on him. Using a glove is less expensive than using a catheter, and turning it inside out prevents powder from getting in the specimen. If the glove overflows, the incontinence pad prevents leakage.

Tina Marks, RN, MS

Specimen trap

For those times when you need to catheterize a patient to get a urine specimen but the urine doesn't flow, try this: Pinch off or clamp the catheter before removing it. This creates a vacuum and traps a small amount of urine in the catheter. Then simply unpinch or unclamp the catheter to release the specimen into your container.

Eugene Heyden, RN

Sterile sample from vesicostomy

When taking a urine sample from a vesicostomy, try this method: Wearing sterile gloves, remove the stoma bag and wafer and clean the area. Using sterile scissors, cut about 4" of a rubber catheter and insert that portion of the catheter into the stoma. Then insert a smaller catheter (such as a #5 French feeding tube) through the first catheter. The urine will drain through the smaller catheter directly into a sterile collection cup. (To speed up urine flow, ask the patient to turn his head away from the stoma and cough.)

Using this technique to collect urine from a vesicostomy will reduce the risk of contamination. It will also ensure accurate urine testing.

Carol Zendehdel, RN, BSN

Stool collection

To obtain stool specimens for guaiac tests from patients with bathroom privileges, give them filter paper instead of toilet paper and a stool cup to hold the paper when used. Most patients find this an easier and less offensive method of collecting stool.

Lillian Plodquist, LPN

A specimen problem

Recently, my mother underwent some diagnostic tests that involved collecting stool specimens at home, then sending them to the laboratory for analysis. When she complained about the difficulty and unpleasantness of collecting the specimens, I thought of a way to make it easier for her.

I suggested that she drape a

piece of plastic wrap over the toilet bowl (with the lid up), keeping the plastic above the water. Then I suggested she tape the sides of the plastic to the outside of the bowl. The stool would fall onto the plastic wrap, which she could easily lift off the toilet to get the specimen. The remainder of the stool could be flushed away and the wrap placed in a bag for disposal.

Brenda Owens, RN

Dry labels for specimen

When you're collecting a 24-hour urine specimen, place the collection jar in a basin that contains a plastic bag filled with ice. That way, the label on the jar will stay dry and the specimen will be cool. Loosely knot the end of the bag so you can refill it as the ice melts.

Loretta A. Debus, RN

Specimen on ice

To keep a specimen iced for transport, prepare a container by following these steps. First, fill a plastic cup (a drinking cup or something larger) and a test tube with water. Place the test tube in the cup and freeze them together. After they're frozen, twist the test tube to remove it. Then you can put the specimen in its place.

This technique is useful for transporting a specimen from the patient's home to the hospital laboratory.

Evelyn H. Lenihan, RN

Containing lab specimens

At the medical center where I work, we place each lab specimen in a reclosable plastic bag and attach the requisition slip to the outside of the bag. This protects us from possible contamination caused by leakage and prevents cross-contamination of specimens.

B. Wilson, LPN

Keeping track of specimens

Here's an easy way to make sure you've collected the right number of stool specimens. Mark what you are collecting on the disposable plastic hat you place on the toilet (for example, "stool specimens x 3"). Then write the number of specimens you need under this (#1, #2, #3); mark off each one as you collect it. Attach a sign to the bathroom door indicating which patient is having the specimens collected.

Tracy Reinert, RN

Securing tubes and drainage sets

Easy way to tape an ET tube

When taping an endotracheal (ET) tube, try attaching a tongue depressor to each end of the tape, then sliding the tape and tongue depressor under the patient's neck. Once the tape is in place, remove the tongue depressors and secure the tape to the patient's face and the ET tube.

The tape won't bunch up, and you'll be able to place it without repositioning the patient's neck.

Dianna Skavdal, RN, RRT

Neck comfort for trach patients

A soft wrist restraint will keep a tracheostomy patient's neck comfortable and will absorb perspiration. I cut the ties off each end of a restraint and make small cuts about 1" apart along its midsection. I thread the trach tie through these holes, then place the restraint around the back of the patient's neck and pull the trach ties through the trach collar.

Lourdes Montano-Maulit, RN

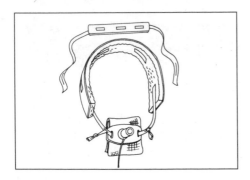

Dry dressing

If your patient has constant leakage around cystostomy tubes, use half a toddler-sized disposable diaper as a dressing. The diaper's liner draws wetness away from the patient's skin, and its outer layer of plastic protects his clothing. Put extra padding inside the dressing if needed. Tape around the edges keeps the dressing in place for 2 days.

Joann Tervenski, RN, BS

Helpful gastrostomy device

I use a stoma wafer and collection bag to prevent excoriation at the site of a leaking gastrostomy tube. I thread the tube through the hole I make in the stoma wafer before attaching the wafer to the site. Then I bring the gastrostomy tube through the bag, secure the bag to the wafer, and tape the bag's opening to the tube. This also helps to anchor the gastrostomy tube so it won't be pulled too far into the stomach during peristalsis.

Katherine Cape, LPN

Tent the tube

Drainage that leaks out *around* abdominal sump or gastrostomy tubes causes wet bedclothes and skin irritation.

To prevent this, use a "tented" tube-and-pouch device, which calls for the following procedures:

Obtain a skin barrier (such as karaya gum or Stomahesive), a drainable ostomy pouch with an adhesive backing, and reinforcing tape. In the centers of the barrier and the pouch adhesive, cut openings no more than ¼" larger than the opening in the patient's abdomen.

Now turn the pouch around. Place a piece of tape about 1" lower than the bottom edge of the adhesive on the pouch's other side. Then cut a hole, slightly smaller than the tube diameter, through the tape and pouch.

To apply the barrier, first clean and dry the patient's skin. Then disconnect the suction momentarily, slip the barrier over the tube, and affix the barrier to the patient.

Next, thread the tube through the hole in the pouch adhesive, then out through the tape-reinforced hole on the pouch's other side. Affix the pouch back securely to the skin barrier.

Now return to the pouch front and wrap tape around the tube where it passes through the tape-reinforced hole. Be sure the tape covers the area *between* the tube and pouch hole where drainage could leak. Continue to wrap tape about 4" up the tube. Fasten the end of the pouch as you would with any drain.

Besides sealing the tube opening, this "tented" tube-in-pouch device serves as a splint to reduce tension on the tube. It also allows you to empty and rinse the pouch from the end, without disturbing the taped seal between tube and pouch. As a result, your patient stays drier, cleaner, and more comfortable.

Carleen D. Parlato, RN, ET

Bag it

The drainage collection devices used after surgery can irritate your patient's skin when they're taped on and changed often. To avoid the discomfort of tape, take a 6" piece of stockinette, seal one end to form a bag, and insert the collection device. Then attach the bag to the patient's dressing, or else make a gauze belt to hold the bag in place.

Because the bag stays in place without tape, you can change the collection devices whenever necessary and not worry about hurting your patient.

Louise Sweeten, RN

Holding the drains

I learned this tip from a postoperative mastectomy patient who had two Jackson-Pratt drains. To hold them when she got out of bed, she pinned a heavy-duty reclosable plastic bag to her gown or robe and placed the drains in it.

Pam Kirk, RN, BSN

Draining dry

Ever care for a patient who'd had a ventricular drainage catheter removed? The catheter site on his forehead continues to drain cerebrospinal fluid, requiring dressing changes every 1 to 2 hours.

So improvise a drainage system. Put a sterile, disposable pediatric urine collector over the catheter site and connect the collector's drainage tube to an empty, sterile I.V. bag.

This device not only eliminates a possible source of infection—the wet dressings—but it also serves as a sterile, closed drainage system to measure the cerebrospinal fluid.

Vivian E. Lyons, RN

Secured with strips

Instead of using tape to hold a nasogastric tube in place, I use tincture of benzoin and Steri-Strips. I apply a small amount of benzoin across the bridge of the patient's nose. When it's dry, I wrap the Steri-Strip around the tube and place it over the patient's nose.

The strips not only adhere to the tube securely, but also look better than tape, so the patients appreciate them, too.

Fran Ellis, RN

Tube twist

Whenever you need to clamp a nasogastric tube briefly (for instance, to ambulate the patient,

between feedings, and so forth), use the tube itself as the clamp. Just fold the tubing 6" from the end and insert this folded portion into the opening.

This handy maneuver saves time spent looking for clamps and doesn't strain the tubing with the added weight of a normal clamp.

Debra Schmaltz, RN, BS

Securing an NG tube

A patient's nostrils may be irritated and he may eventually develop skin breakdown when he has a nasogastric (NG) tube. I've devised a simple, inexpensive way to avoid these problems.

Cut a 4" piece of 1"-wide adhesive tape. About 1" from the top, make a ½" deep cut. Then make another ½"-deep cut about 2½" from the top of the tape. Fold this middle section under itself and tab the end. Cut down from the folded section to the end.

Then use a 2" x 2" gauze pad

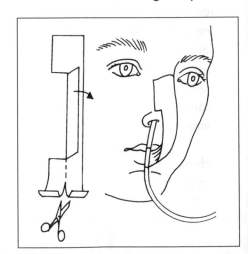

soaked with stoma adhesive to dab the top of the patient's nose. Attach the upper end of the tape to the nose, making sure the wide section is above the nostrils. Wrap the remaining strand around the NG tube and back onto itself.

Now you can see the nostrils, and the NG tube is secure. This method also allows you to anchor a feeding tube at the same time.

Karan R. Quintero, RN, BSN

Tape prep

Before taping a nasogastric tube to a patient's face, wipe the area with a Skin-Prep swab pad. This will remove oil from the skin, so the tape will stick better. Let the invisible residue dry for 30 to 45 seconds before applying tape. (The unpleasant odor will subside when the area is dry.)

Cynthia Mace Mills, RN, MSN

Neat bandage for NG tubes

To stabilize a nasogastric (NG) tube, I place a knuckle bandage vertically on the patient's nose; I attach the bottom to the tube. This will absorb moisture and eliminate the mess of tape. Also, you can easily remove it to change or reposition the tube.

Cynthia Blough, RN

Stuck-up nasogastric tube

When a patient who has many tubes and I.V. lines needs special positioning, the vent port of a Salem sump tube can end up in a dependent position—and so may leak. To keep the vent port in an upright position, I loosely tape it to the main lumen. Then, I make a channel at the top of the headboard by taping a shorter piece of tape to another longer piece. I thread the tube through this channel.

Gail Dittes, RN

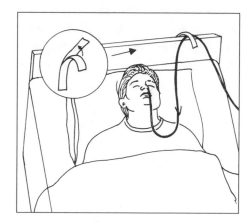

All strapped in

Use Montgomery straps to secure indwelling urinary catheters. First, cut a 4" x 4" section from a Montgomery strap. Then into the section's center, cut two parallel ¼" slits 1" apart. After weaving the string supplied with the strap through the slits, apply the strap's sticky side to the patient and tie the string around the catheter.

This simple device can all but eliminate the need to reposition indwelling catheters. You'll save yourself time and save your patients considerable discomfort.

Jacqueline Kasulanis, RN

Catheter tubing that stays put

When a patient is in a geriatric chair, his catheter drainage tubing may move around. So it may not be in the proper position to drain into the collection bag. I have a solution:

I place two patches of a self-adhesive fastening tape vertically on the side of the chair, just below the armrest. The tubing runs horizontally between the patches, and it's secured with a 3" piece of the adhesive. Then I put the drainage bag in a cloth bag and attach it to the side of the chair, toward the back.

I've found that the catheter tubing stays in place and the drainage bag is hidden from view.

Toni DeRyke, RN

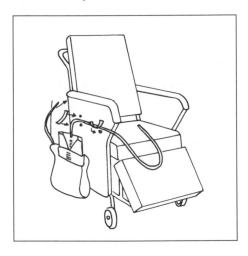

Tapeless tubing tricks

Problem: To stabilize a patient's indwelling urinary catheter, you tape the tubing to his thigh—but the tapes irritate his skin. Solution: Try using a long piece of gauze instead. Wrap the gauze once around the patient's thigh. Lay the tubing over the gauze, then wrap the rest of the gauze around the thigh over the tubing and tape the gauze to itself. Now the tubing is sandwiched between two layers of gauze. To be doubly sure the tubing is secure, tape it to the gauze.

Carol M. Croston, RN

Stress-free catheterization

Here's an easier way to catheterize a spastic multiple sclerosis patient:

Invert an abduction wedge so that the wide end is at the patient's knees. Flex her knees slightly, which will allow her hips to rotate and her feet to come together. Then strap the wedge to her legs.

This technique would also work with other female patients who may not cooperate during catheterization.

Bob Whitlow, LPN

Pajama game

An irrational patient will sometimes risk traumatic injury by pulling on an indwelling urinary catheter.

Discourage this by putting a pajama bottom on the patient and running the tubing down the inside of the pajama leg. Usually, this is so successful that conventional restraints aren't necessary.

E. Rexine Stott, RN

In good form

Instead of trying to stabilize an I.V. line in a pediatric patient's foot with an uncomfortable I.V. board, try making a splint with leftover pieces of Polyform from your hospital's orthopedic department. Polyform is an orthotic plastic that you can heat and mold to the shape of your patient's foot and lower leg. After padding the molded Polyform splint with gauze, put it on the patient and tape it in place. You'll find that the splint stabilizes the I.V. line without causing your patient discomfort.

Jeannine Aucoin, RN

Arterial tubing change

Changing arterial line tubing can be messy if you can't control bleeding from a patient's catheter. And two nurses may be needed to do it.

But you can make this an easy procedure simply by placing a blood pressure cuff above the arterial line site and adding pressure until it's about 20 mm Hg above the patient's systolic pressure. You'll inflate the cuff only during the time you take to switch the tubing.

This pressure slows arterial blood flow so you can quickly and easily change the tubing.

Craig Uhler, RN

Mobile equipment

Setting up for insertion of a pulmonary artery catheter or a tempo-rary pacemaker takes less time if the necessary supplies are readily available. We keep the supplies for these procedures in two small, stainless steel carts with wheels. When we need the supplies, we simply roll the cart into the patient's room.

Jeanne Logue-Hunter, RN

Applying dressings, bandages, and compresses

Dressed for comfort

Here's a way to minimize painful dressing changes when a patient has a burn or abrasion: Apply the ointment on the non-adhering dressing instead of the wound. Then lay the dressing over the wound.

Tom Little, RN

Painless dressing

To ease the pain of dressing changes for patients who have had nose surgery, I devised a convenient procedure. First, I cut a piece of 1"-wide Kerlix gauze, about 25" long, and tape the ends together. Then I twist it in the middle, making a large figure eight, and place a 2" x 2" gauze pad in the middle.

To apply the dressing, I hook one loop around each of the patient's ears and center the gauze on his nose. Changing the dressing is simple: I just unhook one loop and replace the gauze. No tape touches the patient's sensitive skin.

Peggy Holden, RN

Inventive dressings

We recently cared for a patient who had high bilateral leg amputations—and dressings that just wouldn't stay in place, no matter what kind of bandages we used over them. Every time we turned him, the dressings came off and we had to replace them.

Finally we tried a pair of women's long-line underpants (the kind that almost reach the knee) to keep the dressings in place—and it worked. We stitched each leg of the underpants closed, curving the seam so that it conformed to the patient's stumps. We opened the middle seam to make room for an indwelling urinary catheter and to allow the patient to use a bedpan. Then we applied some Velcro at the waistband. With a pair of these underpants worn over his dressings, the patient could be moved without trouble.

Hazel L. Shaw, RN

A net worth of comfort

If you're caring for a patient who has a wound on his hips or buttocks, here's a way to hold the dressing in place without tape: Use a large-sized, tubular, stretchy, net material. Just cut the length of material you need, then pull it over the patient's feet and up over his hips. This will hold the patient's dressing securely in place—without irritating his skin.

Danalee Nelson, RN

Patchwork

In the doctor's office where I work, minor surgical procedures are performed routinely. Applying dressings to irregularly shaped or hard-to-reach wounds (such as those behind the ear or over the coccyx) is always a challenge. I've found that small, flexible oval eye patches can be applied easily and securely to these wounds.

Kathy Smernoff, LVN

Double-duty strap

I work on an orthopedics unit and care for many patients who have had total knee replacements. The knee exerciser they use comes with a Velcro strap. We've found the strap also works well to stabilize a patient's leg when it's elevated or when he's sitting in a wheelchair.

Kathy Meyer, RN

Wrap and roll

Applying an elastic bandage to a patient's leg can be a one-person job if you do it this way: Use an unwrapped roll of toilet paper as a footrest for the patient. This will lift the patient's leg far enough off the bed so you can easily wrap the leg without needing someone else to hold it.

Jean Kindle, RN

Other plaster problems

Always use cold water for easy removal of plaster from patients and instruments after a cast has been applied. If you get plaster on your uniform, let the plaster dry, then brush it off.

Because working with plaster can dry your hands, keep a bottle of hand lotion nearby and use it frequently.

Let mothers soak the serial casts off their babies. And add a little vinegar to the water to aid removal of the casts.

Elsie Hajdics, RN

No fallout here

Bulky dressings on large or draining abdominal wounds sometimes slip off when patients get out of bed. To avoid this problem, apply Montgomery straps in the conventional manner, that is, two straps affixed vertically along the wound. Then place a third, smaller, Montgomery strap horizontally below the other straps and lace it through the vertical straps' lower holes. The horizontal strap keeps the dressings in place so the patient can move about confidently.

Constance J. Gramzow, RN, BSN

A toe hold

If a patient needs a warm compress on his toe, use a disposable glove to keep the compress in place and his bed dry. After applying the compress, slip the glove over the patient's toes and lower part of his foot. The glove keeps the compress from getting the bed wet and maintains the warmth longer.

Pam Miller, LPN

Caring for skin and wounds

Unmasked

When administering oxygen by mask to postanesthesia room patients who have had nasal reconstructive surgery, we cut off the upper portion of the mask. This keeps the mask from touching the patient's nose but still ensures that he receives oxygen.

Marci Smith, RN

Perspiration pickup

Keeping electrocardiogram leads on a diaphoretic patient can be difficult. So I spray a small amount of antiperspirant on a clean, dry washcloth, then wipe it on the patient's skin where I want the leads to adhere. The antiperspirant keeps the skin dry, so the leads stay in place.

Ralph Gonzalez, RN

Protecting skin from electrodes

The electrodes used for continuously monitoring an electrocardiogram (ECG) can cause skin breakdown. Here's what I do to prevent it: I place the ECG electrode on the nonsticky side of a hydrocolloid dressing and cut around the electrode to form a patch. Then I cut a small hole in the center of the dressing to expose the conductive gel. Finally, I remove the protective film from the sticky side of the dressing and place the dressing on clean, dry skin.

This method will protect the patient's skin without interfering with ECG tracings.

Debra J. Gardill, RN, CCRN

Covering pacemaker wires

We routinely care for patients with pacemaker wires. The wires are taped to the patient's abdomen, so we had to come up with a way to keep the tips of the wires aseptic. We solved the problem by protecting the tips with rubber needle cov-

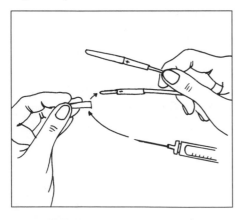

ers from syringes. They fit snugly and don't irritate the patient's skin.

Judy Gilmore, RN

Loose hair: Sticky solution

After you prep a body area for surgery, loose hairs can be a problem. So I towel-dry the area after shaving, then use a long piece of 3" adhesive tape to pick up any loose hair on the skin gently. Of course, I use this procedure only for patients with good skin turgor.

Linda B. Harris, RN

Comforting cushion

To prevent skin breakdown in elderly patients who have spinal deformities, we cushion their bony prominences with sanitary pads when they're sitting down. For patients with arm slings, we wrap a long maternity pad in a disposable washcloth and place it under the strap around their necks.

Valrie Loftes, LPN

Socks under splints

A patient with arthritis or carpal tunnel syndrome who must wear a wrist splint may suffer skin irritation or breakdown under the splint. But you can prevent this with a pair of cotton knee socks.

Cut off the toe portion and make a hole in the heel of each sock. Slip the sock over the patient's hand; put his thumb through the hole in the heel, his fingers through the cutoff toe. Then apply the splint.

The cotton absorbs perspiration better than knit material or a stockinette. And if you make two protectors from one pair of socks, the patient will always have one to wear while the other's being washed.

Beverly Walking, RN

The right touch

Here's a gentle way to apply ointments or lotions to sore and tender skin.

When you put on your latex gloves, leave some space at the tips of your fingers to trap air; then use them to apply the ointment. The air-filled tips will feel soft to the patient, allowing you to touch his skin without causing discomfort.

Ruth B. Pratt, RN

Ointment applicator

Add a disposable syringe (minus the needle) to your weapons for fighting decubitus ulcers. Remove the syringe plunger, squeeze ointment into the syringe barrel, and replace the plunger. After cleaning the ulcer as ordered, squirt the ointment onto the ulcer. The pencil-thin ointment lines will allow you to target each crevice and fold.

Lynda L. Scherff, LPN

Tick pick

To remove a tick from a patient's skin, cover the tick with petroleum jelly. After a few minutes, the tick

will suffocate and you can remove it painlessly with forceps.

Linda DeLuca, RN, BSN

Peel-off splinters

I've found an easy way to remove splinters or cactus spines that are embedded in a patient's skin. Apply a layer of gel facial mask to the skin and let it dry. When you peel off the gel, the splinters will come with it. Because the gel is made for skin, it shouldn't irritate the patient. Plus, there's no sticky residue.

Marie Christopher, BSN

No-drop irrigation

Cancer patients can get shallow excoriated lesions from radiation therapy. Daily irrigation with equal parts of hydrogen peroxide and sterile water can be cold and messy for the patient—when you use traditional irrigating equipment. So try using a sterilized spray bottle instead—the kind used for spray-on glass cleaner. You can deliver an adequate amount of solution, with a minimum of dripping and a maximum of comfort for your patient.

Joann Tervenski, RN, BS

Eliminating messy irrigation

Using a shampoo rinse tray that has a drainage tube, I've found that I can irrigate a wound with minimal discomfort for the patient—and less mess.

First, I put disposable underpads beneath the patient for extra protection. Then I elevate the area of the body I want to irrigate on an inflatable, plastic doughnut ring, with the rinse tray under it. As I irrigate the wound, the excess drainage flows from the tray, through the drainage tube, and into a container that's at the bedside.

Mary Ellen Dorsey, RN

Prelude to wound care

I've found a painless way to clean dirt and grease from the surrounding skin before doing wound care. Soak a cotton swab or 2" x 2" gauze pad in mineral oil and gently rub the grease from the patient's skin, carefully avoiding the wound. Then gently scrub the skin with diluted surgical scrub soap (1 part soap to 3 parts water or saline). Rinse with sterile water or normal saline solution. Now you're ready to proceed with wound care.

Pauline Reaburn, RN, BSN, MEd

Delicate removal

To clean dried blood from sensitive skin, apply a generous amount of K-Y jelly and allow time for it to soften the blood. Then carefully wipe it off.

Vickie Milton, RN, BSN

Tarnished injuries

Some patients who come to the emergency department where I work have injuries covered with grease or tar. To remove the grease or tar without causing more pain or trauma, we gently wipe it off with gauze or cotton balls soaked in mineral oil. The oil cuts through the grease or tar quickly; then we can easily remove the oil with a liquid soap.

Kathleen Rohrer, RN

Painless removal of paint

To remove oil-based paint from the body, most people think first of using the solvent, turpentine. All well and good, but turpentine cannot be used around the eyes or mouth, for it can irritate and hurt. That doesn't help matters, especially with children, who are apt to have wiped their eyes with paint-covered hands anyway.

To solve this problem, use mineral oil. It's nonirritating and effectively removes paint.

Patricia L. Badowski, RN

Particle picker

When accident victims come to our emergency department covered with small glass particles, we remove the glass with our wall suction unit. We turn the unit on to medium or low and gently pass the suction tubing over the glass-covered area. Afterward, we throw away the tubing and carefully clean out the suction bottle.

Jerry Taylor, LPN

It's oil for the better #2

You can use mineral oil (or baby oil) to remove fiberglass fibers from a patient's skin. Soak a cotton ball with the oil and coat the affected area. Then gently wipe the area with a terry-cloth towel to remove the fibers and ease irritation.

Susan Boisvert, LPN, SN

Vacuum cleaning

In the emergency department where I work, we use a hand-held, rechargeable vacuum cleaner to remove stones and dirt from patients' wounds. We also use it to remove glass particles from patients' skin, hair, and clothes without contaminating wounds or causing further injury.

Tom G. Bartol, RN

Effective seal for punctures

When an unhealed puncture site is leaking after an abdominal paracentesis, here's what I do to prevent infection: First, I position the patient on his back. Using sterile technique, I clean the area. Then I dab it with dry sections of an absorbable gelatin sponge holding each section on the site for several minutes. When the oozing stops, I apply collodion. I keep the patient in that position for about 10 minutes. Remember to get a doctor's order before doing this procedure.

Sylvia Hodin, RN, OCN

A spirited cleanup

After removing a patient's cast, we wipe his skin with alcohol. The alcohol removes any dead skin and dirt that has accumulated under the cast, and it refreshes the skin as well. If the patient's skin is dry, we follow up with skin cream or lotion.

Connie Mongar, RN
Lisa Schill, LPN

Sting stuff

If you find yourself treating a lot of insect bites and stings, stock up on some Benylin cough syrup and Maalox. Just mix a small amount of the cough syrup with the Maalox and spread the mixture over the bite or sting area. It cuts down itching and pain and is soothing and cooling, too.

Jeannette Raschke, RN, BSN

Bath-time bolster

To keep skin pampered, pour some baby lotion into the water before bathing a patient. This eliminates the need to apply lotion after washing and drying (which patients appreciate if they're on complete bed rest). Also, baby lotion is an inexpensive substitute for bath oil. Diaphoretic patients especially will appreciate this.

Christy K. Greco, LPN

Blow-dry skin treatment

An extremely obese patient's deep folds of flesh present a real skin-care problem. After his bath, it's difficult to get the skin between these folds completely dry. As a result, the skin may break down.

To solve the problem, use a hair blow-dryer. To be safe, set the dryer on a low speed and always keep it moving. Test the airflow with your hand as well to make sure the patient's skin doesn't get too hot.

Besides preventing further skin breakdown, the blow-dry treatment gives the patient's medicated skin creams and powders a chance to work and keeps them from caking together.

Janet S. Ford, RN

Preferred powder

Often, patients in our critical care units who are receiving steroids or have diabetes develop a yeast infection in the groin or under a pendulous breast. We apply powder to these areas to reduce moisture buildup and increase comfort.

But we've found that a cornstarch powder seems to make the infection worse, because the cornstarch and moisture from the skin act as a medium for yeast growth. Talcum powder, on the other hand, has a mineral base and doesn't promote yeast growth.

Doris K. Putland, RN, CCRN

Healing powder

Try this solution for treating excoriated skin caused by chronic diar-

rhea. Mix 9 parts cornstarch with 1 part boric acid powder. Clean the affected area, then shake the powder on. (We use large, clean salt or pepper shakers.) The powder dries the skin, helps it heal, and also seems to prevent yeast infections.

Our nursing staff has been so pleased with the results of this treatment that our hospital pharmacy mixes the powder for us. We encourage the patient's family to continue the treatment after discharge.

Debbie Bornholdt, RN, BSN

A leak-proof bag

Sometimes patients undergoing peritoneal dialysis have a problem with dialysate leaking onto their skin around the catheter insertion site. We solve this problem by cleaning the skin, applying a Stomahesive wafer around the insertion site, and applying a colostomy bag on top of the wafer. We then pass the catheter through the bottom opening of the bag. Finally, we wrap rubber bands around the bottom of the bag and tubing to make it secure. The colostomy bag traps leaking dialysate and protects the patient's skin.

Nancy L. Eder, RN

Rings on their fingers

Want to know a simple trick for getting a ring off a swollen finger?

Use a few feet of string or silk suture. Slip one end under the ring. Beginning next to the distal edge of the ring, wind the other end of the string toward the fingertip. The windings should be close together to prevent the swollen tissue from bulging through. With the coils of string tightly in place, take the short end of the string on the proximal side of the ring and pull it toward the tip of the finger. This pulls the ring off over the unwinding coil.

Evangeline Goodway, RN

Arm pads

When a patient has to wear an arm splint for a long time, he could develop pressure ulcers or skin breakdown. To prevent such skin problems, pad the splint with disposable sanitary minipads. The pads cushion the skin, absorb perspiration, and are inexpensive to replace.

Christine Destro, RN

Breast support for mastectomy patient

A patient recovering from a unilateral mastectomy will probably feel better if her remaining breast has some support. But a bra may irritate the sensitive sutured area. You can solve this problem by cutting off the bra's unneeded cup and shoulder strap. The other cup, elastic band, and fasteners are left for comfortable support without irritating the sutures.

Marie M. Savoie, BSN

Skin saver

Besides being painful, frequent dressing changes can irritate sensitive or frail skin. So I cut strips of DuoDERM about 1" to 2" wide and slightly longer than the wound. I prep the patient's skin with benzoin, then place the strips of DuoDERM on each side of the wound.

Next, I place the dressing over the wound and cover it with tape so that the tape adheres only to the DuoDERM. Finally, I fold back the edges of the tape; I can gently remove the tape from the DuoDERM at the next dressing change.

This method works really well because the DuoDERM adheres to the benzoin on the skin and helps prevent tape burns. Plus, the patient's skin integrity isn't compromised.

Jennifer L. O'Brien, RN, BSN

Foot care for the elderly

If an elderly patient has toe contractures, you might have difficulty giving him proper foot care. Here's what I do to solve the problem:

I clean his toes with a disposable, sponge-tipped toothbrush. A toothbrush easily fits between the toes without having to spread them apart. I dry the skin after cleaning

and apply powder as ordered.
This procedure works well, and it's
comfortable for the patient.

J. Kelly, LPN

Cotton for comfort

If latex gloves irritate your skin, buy a
pair of cotton gloves to wear underneath them. The gloves will protect
your skin, and you can even use hand
lotion before you put them on.

Kaye Horrigan, RN

Team up against decubiti

To prevent decubiti—and to treat
them when they occur—
Maimonides Hospital Geriatric
Center, Montreal, Quebec, uses a
team approach.

The nursing coordinator and the
infection-surveillance nurse helped
form a decubiti control team that
includes themselves, an in-service
educator, a doctor, a dietitian, and a
physiotherapist.

The team meets twice a month
to review data compiled by the
infection-surveillance nurse. Team
members then make rounds to
assess the patients, their nutritional
status, and the treatment plans. The
team recommends changes in the
patients' diets and the treatment
plans as needed, and the staff nurses
incorporate the recommendations
into their care plans and document
them on the patients' charts.
Besides the usual means of treating
decubiti, the team also recommends

nonnursing techniques that may be
helpful, for example, ultrasonogra-
phy or infrared treatment.

When the center first started
using the team approach 3 years
ago, most of the decubiti the nursing staff reported had already pro-
gressed to tissue loss. Now the
nurses are reporting when they first
spot a reddened area. Because
decubiti are reported and treated
earlier, healing time has been
reduced; in most cases, ulcers that
used to take months to heal now
heal within a single month.

Margaret Bougie, RN, BSN
Judy Seri, RN

8 I.V. Therapy

Clean up before venipuncture

When you need to clip hair from a patient's arm before performing a venipuncture, remove residual hair with a piece of 2" or 3"-wide paper tape. Touch the adhesive side of the tape to the site several times to pick up hairs that could later cause infection. You might also try this to remove hair from a patient's sheets and pillow case.

Cindy Mauldin, RN

Tabs to grab

Before starting an I.V., cut the tape you'll need and turn under the ends on each piece. This will create tabs that won't stick to your gloves during the procedure.

Deb Falk, RN

Illuminating a vein

If you have to insert an I.V. catheter but you can't see or feel the vein, try using a penlight. Wipe both the patient's skin and the bulb end of the penlight with alcohol. Turn on the penlight and place it on the patient's skin. Look directly in front of the beam—you should see the vein. Turn off the penlight and insert the catheter as usual.

Terrilynn M. Quillen, RN

I.V.s in the bag

Our emergency department is always stocked with various kinds of I.V. start kits. We make them ourselves, using self-locking plastic bags filled with the following supplies:
- I.V. solution
- I.V. tubing
- I.V. angiocath
- Tourniquet
- Alcohol wipe
- Bandage
- Antibiotic ointment
- ½" tape

In an emergency, the I.V. bags save us time trying to find the supplies we need.

Eileen M. Suraci, RN

Teaching first

Before performing venipuncture, consider patient teaching your first priority. Ask your patient if he's had an I.V. before. Tell him why he needs it, how venipuncture is done, and how much discomfort he'll feel.

Do your best to appear self-confident. Remember, patient anxiety can trigger vasoconstriction, making venipuncture more difficult for you and more painful for him.

Doris A. Millam, RN, CRNI, MS

Squeezercise

If you have a patient with poor veins who needs frequent I.V. therapy, here's a simple exercise program to build up those veins:

Have the patient squeeze a small rubber ball in each hand as often as possible every day. In a few weeks, veins should protrude above the dorsal surface of the patient's hands, making the I.V. insertion much easier and less painful.

Jay M. Davis, MD, PhD

Marking the vessel

Palpating a vein or artery is difficult while wearing gloves. So I find the blood vessel first, mark it lightly with my fingernail, then put on gloves to do the venipuncture or arterial puncture. The mark I've made shows me where the vessel is, and it also lets the patient know how the needle stick will feel.

Ann Marie Dente-Cassidy, RN, CCRN, MSN

A sticky problem

When starting an I.V. on a patient in isolation, you wear sterile gloves, of course. But the gloves may cause some problems.

For instance, the tape on the I.V. site can easily stick to the gloves instead of your patient's arm, and if you move your hand away, the I.V. could pull out.

To prevent this, wrap tape around each of your middle three fingers over your gloves before you begin taping the I.V. in place. The tape on the I.V. site won't stick to your gloves as readily as before, the I.V. will stay put, and you—and your patient—won't have to worry about reinserting the I.V.

Terri Stambaugh, RN

No-mess I.V.

When I start an I.V., I place a 2" x 2" piece of gauze under the I.V. hub. This prevents blood from dripping on my gloves, body, or the floor when I remove the needle—the gauze is there to catch it.

Chris Lotti, RN, BSN

I.D. for I.V. infusions

When I start an I.V. infusion, I remove part of the catheter package label stating the brand, length, and gauge size. Then I write the date, the time, and my initials on the label and tape it to the I.V. dressing. This eliminates confusion if any problems arise.

Marianne Morissette, RN, BSN

Intermittent-infusion device: Combining steps

In our unit, we often have patients who need an intermittent-infusion lock cap applied to a catheter. Before inserting the catheter, I spike the rubber tip of the cap with a needle attached to a 3-ml saline-filled syringe. After the catheter is in the vein, I remove the tourniquet, place a 2" x 2" piece of gauze under the catheter hub, and withdraw the catheter needle. Finally, I connect the intermittent-infusion device cap (with the needle and syringe) to the hub, aspirate for blood, and flush with the saline. You can also flush with heparin (if it's hospital policy). Remove the gauze; then dress according to policy.

Janie Cook, RN

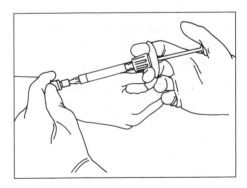

Reducing skin tears

Before starting an I.V. infusion on an elderly patient, we wrap a 1" x 6" piece of foam around his arm. (We've found that foam packaged in some angiosets is the right size.) We tape the foam to the patient's arm so only 1" of tape at both ends touches the skin. Then we can tape the I.V. tubing to the foam. When we remove the tape on the tubing, we don't tear sensitive skin.

Joyce Nelson, RN, BSN

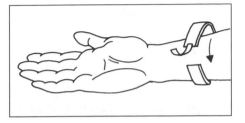

No-stick blood sample

When a patient who's undergoing thrombolytic therapy doesn't have an arterial line in place, we insert a 16-gauge catheter into a median vein, then attach an extension set with a T extender and a 3-way stopcock to the catheter. We connect the I.V. tubing to the stopcock. When necessary, we can draw blood from the stopcock and avoid sticking the patient.

Margery Lebel, RN, CCRN

Administration

Milking an I.V.

When an I.V. infusion slows to less than the desired flow rate, you could spend a lot of time trying to flush it. Instead, try this first: Open and close the roller clamp several times on a section of the tube that hasn't been clamped. This milking action will often return the I.V. to its normal flow rate. Of course, make sure there are no other signs of infiltration or occlusion before trying this technique.

Myron Tassin, RN, BSN

The light touch

If you suspect I.V. infiltration in a patient with difficult veins, turn on a flashlight and hold it against his skin, directly over the suspicious site.

If I.V. fluid has infiltrated into the tissue, the beam will highlight the size of the infiltration. If no fluid has infiltrated, only a small halo will appear around the flashlight.

Using this trick can save you from having to do extra checks. Then, if necessary, you can stop the I.V. before the infiltration gets worse.

Betty Woodfin, RN

Pushing medications into the right port

A critically ill patient will probably have multiple I.V. lines and drug infusions. Here's a way to make sure bolus medications aren't pushed into the wrong I.V. line.

Write "push port" on a piece of tape, then place the tape around the injection port in the I.V. line that isn't being used for continuous drug infusions.

This will flag the port that should be used for push medications, which is especially important in an emergency.

Gwen Avila, RN, CCRN

A real loosener

Have you ever tried to loosen I.V. tubing or a distal port connector with a hemostat? If so, you know how easily the hemostat could slip and cause damage. Instead, use a flat tourniquet. Just wrap the tourniquet around the tubing or connector that needs to be loosened and twist. A tourniquet also works well in loosening tight lids on medication bottles.

Bonnie Forbes, RN

No more tangled tubing

If a patient needs a certain medication infused at regular intervals, we leave his I.V. tubing hanging so it's readily available. But the tubing could get tangled, so we clip a small plastic clothespin between the distal end of the tubing and the needle

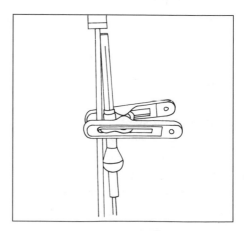

cap, then attach the clothespin to the tubing. The needle cap won't fall off because the clothespin is holding the needle upright. You can use clothespins of the same color for all of the patient's medications.

After the patient is discharged, you don't have to throw away the clothespins; they're reusable if they're disinfected first. Soak them in a 10% bleach solution to avoid cross-contamination.

Dorothy M. Huebener, RN

No more kinks

Here's what I do to prevent a multi-lumen catheter from kinking: I cut a straw to the desired length, then split it lengthwise. I place the tubing in the straw, then lightly tape over the split to keep the straw in place. Because the straw encases the tubing, it prevents kinks. This procedure also works well on feeding tubes.

Sonja Jones, RN

Hang-up for I.V. bags

In the emergency clinic where I work, we use L-shaped wall hangers (the kind used for plants) to hang I.V. bags. This way, we don't have to move I.V. poles in and out of small areas. Patients who have I.V.s at home can also use this tip.

K. Nippes, RN, CCRN

Positioning the pump

If I'm caring for an ambulatory patient who's receiving I.V. solutions through a pump, I place the pump at or below chest level on the I.V. pole. The pole is easier to push and it's less likely to fall over if the base hits an object.

April Spectrum, RN

Maintenance

Clamp that won't crack tubing

Catheters and I.V. tubing can crack when they're clamped with a hemostat. I place a rubber needle cap over each tine of the hemostat—the caps pad the teeth, so the catheter or tubing won't crack. I've also found that the caps provide a firmer grip when I'm using the hemostat to loosen luer-lock hubs.

Ruby L. Baker, RN, BSN

Ring around the I.V. tubing

When an intensive care unit patient has multiple I.V. lines, the tubing can get caught in the side rail or become tangled as he moves. To prevent this, I attach a shower-curtain ring to the side rail and place all the I.V. tubing through it. The patient can move around more freely, and I don't have to worry about I.V. tubing.

Mary Lu Morris, RN, BSN

Securing multiple lines

Multiple-lumen catheters can be hard to secure, and I.V. tubing can easily become tangled. You could tape the lumens or tubing to the patient's skin, but that may cause excoriation. Here's what I do instead:

I take a tabbed device used for indwelling urinary catheters (such as Cath-Secure), remove the paper backing, and place it on the patient's shoulder. I put the lumens or the tubing between the pieces of Velcro on the tab, then fold the tab over. The lumens or tubing will be held securely without irritating the patient's skin. Dressing and ambulating the patient will be easier too.

Susan Stewart, LPN

Label reminder

Here's a way to ensure that I.V. tubing is labeled when it's changed: Attach a peel-off label to each box of I.V. tubing. When you change the tubing, just place the label on it and write the date and time.

Doris A. Millam, RN, CRNI, MS

Weight until the calm

The thrashing and pulling of confused, combative patients sometimes necessitates restarting I.V. lines several times. So, after establishing an I.V., place a 5-lb sandbag under a standard arm board. Then wrap the sandbag, arm board, and arm with an elastic bandage. The weight of the sandbag, which can be varied as needed, keeps the arm immobile.

Ann Hensley, LPN

A secure I.V. catheter

Securing an I.V. catheter on a diaphoretic patient or a patient in a mist tent can be difficult. Because of the moisture, the tape doesn't stick and the catheter can dislodge.

But if I prepare the patient's skin with a thin coat of liquid adhesive, the tape will remain secure. The catheter will also stay in place, and the liquid adhesive will protect the patient's skin from irritation.

Chris Scheer, RN, BSN

Gentle reminder

To remind a patient not to bend his hand or wrist when he has an I.V. inserted, try this: Cover a peripad with a washcloth, and tape the covered peripad to the patient's palm and forearm. This makes a soft, non-bulky arm board—a subtle reminder to the patient to keep his wrist or hand straight.

Lou Ann Jeffries, RN

Boxed boards

If an I.V. arm board isn't available when you need one, just tape a washcloth or small towel around the empty I.V. tubing box and use that instead. The long, narrow box makes an excellent temporary I.V. arm board and saves you time looking for the real thing.

Carol Kenck Crispin, RN, MEd

Protected port

To stabilize a heparin lock in an active patient, use an eye bubble. After inserting the catheter and applying the dressing, tape the eye bubble over the infusion port and tubing. The clear plastic bubble protects the lock from accidental jostling, yet allows you to see the port. To inject medication into the port, just peel back the tape and remove the bubble. Replace the bubble when the medication is infused.

Lorrie Tatman, RN

Heparin lock(ed) in place

A heparin lock is inserted at such an angle that it may protrude and become dislodged. To remedy this, fill the space between the heparin lock and the patient's arm with some cotton or gauze. Place a piece of tape over the lock, leaving only the rubber port exposed. Now, no matter how active the patient is, the lock won't become dislodged.

Kathie M. Olney, RN

Drawing blood with a vacuum

When using a winged-tip needle set for a venipuncture, try putting a heparin lock cap on the open end of the tubing. Then, when you see the flashback of blood in the tubing, insert the vacutainer needle into the heparin cap. The vacuum will draw blood through the tubing into the collection tube. You can fill many tubes using this technique.

John E. Elsner, RN

Syringes attached

When I prepare my I.V. medication solutions, I tape a 1 ½- to 2-ml syringe of saline solution to every I.V. medication bag I hang. This reminds me to flush out the heparin lock before I start the I.V. medication.

Theresa Tucker, RN

Shower cap

Make showering easier for a patient who has a heparin lock: Cut off four of the fingers (but not the thumb) from a plastic glove. Pull the glove over the patient's hand and wrist, covering the heparin lock with the thumb portion of the glove. Cover the insertion and dressing site with the rest of the glove and tape the ends of the glove to the patient's skin. The glove keeps the site dry and is easier to apply than plastic wrap.

Ann Damore, RN, BSN

Disconnection protection

Before disconnecting I.V. tubing, I place an alcohol swab under the hub of the catheter and the old tubing. Then I attach the new tubing. The swab absorbs any I.V. fluid drip and blood return. It also protects the new connector from contamination by normal skin flora.

Linda C. LeVee, RN

Quick fix for cracked port

Here's a way to fix a cracked side port on a central venous line introducer temporarily until it can be changed: Insert a 14-gauge over-the-needle catheter into the lumen and remove the needle. This will prevent air from entering the vessel, fluid from leaking out, and the lumen from clotting. Now you can use the port.

Mary E. Hodges, RN, C, CCRN, MS

MEDICATIONS

Preparation

Handy storage in a floss caddy

Here's a way to organize and store medication vials and ampules on units that don't routinely have storage containers: Put them in large plastic embroidery floss caddies, the kind you can find in craft stores.

I label each interior section with the name of the medication, then place a corresponding name label on the outside lid of the caddy. So the medications are easily located and conveniently stored.

Regina Schuch, RN, CGC, BSN

Planning ahead

When an active patient is receiving intermittent piggyback medications through a heparin lock, I post a dosage schedule where he can see it. That way, he'll know when he'll be less mobile, and he can plan his daily activities accordingly.

Sharon Richer, RN

A schooling in organization

I'm a school nurse who must keep track of many students' medications—those taken daily and as needed. To do this, I use a plastic, 42-drawer cabinet usually found in workshops to hold screws, nuts, and bolts. I put each student's medication container or inhaler and folded permit form in a different drawer of the cabinet. Then I label each drawer with the student's name, medication, and dose using different-colored labels for daily and p.r.n. medications. I keep the drawers in alphabetical order.

Lorraine L. Lemus, RN

Drug administration: Ready reference

I tied a spiral-bound medication reference book to our medication cart. This way, we always have the book at our fingertips when we need it.

Jacqueline Zabresky, RN, CCRN

Safe storage for medication

Before discharging a patient, you should discuss not only the proper dosage for his medications, but also *where* he'll store them. Make sure he knows that he shouldn't keep them in the bathroom because moisture from the shower or tub could alter the drugs' potency. Tell him that he should store the medications in his bedroom—out of his children's or grandchildren's reach.

Sylvia T. Joseph, RN

Eyedrop reminder

When caring for patients with cardiac problems, be sure to question them about *all* medications they're taking, including eyedrops. Ophthalmic timolol maleate (Timoptic), for example, can cause cardiac complications in some patients.

Linda Vasquez, RN

Making medication tasteless

If your patient dislikes the taste of his medication, tell him to suck on some ice for a few moments before you administer it. The ice will numb his taste buds so the medication will go down much easier.

Valerie Rubin Walsh, RN, BSN

Pleasing to the palate

I mix fruit-flavored powdered laxatives with milk shakes, instant breakfast or diet drinks, nonalcoholic eggnog, and yogurt. Because these drinks are thicker than juice or water, they make drinking the laxative more palatable.

Anita J. Rider, RN

Medication refrigeration

Store aluminum hydroxide (Amphojel) in the refrigerator. When the medication's cool, it doesn't leave a chalky sensation in the patient's mouth. Also, the patient seems more aware of the drug's cool temperature than of its unpleasant flavor.

Penny Pica, RN

Tasteful lozenge

To make clotrimazole (Mycelex) lozenges more palatable for patients who have oral candidiasis, try adding peppermint flavoring. After removing the needle, fill a tuberculin syringe with 0.25 to 0.50 ml of flavoring (available in grocery stores). Put the lozenge in a medicine cup and coat it with 3 or 4 drops of flavoring.

Allison A. Fontenot, RN, BSN

Syringe versus spoon

Oral antibiotics are prescribed for many of the babies brought to an emergency department. The nurse usually administers the first dose, using a syringe to squirt the medication into the baby's mouth, then gives the baby's mother the prescription for the remaining doses. But if the baby needs a second dose during the night—before the mother can get to a pharmacy—give her a single dose to take home.

A disposable syringe makes an ideal container for a single dose of oral medication. When you give the initial dose, show the mother how to use the syringe safely.

E. Rogers, RN

Let them down easy

If a patient has difficulty swallowing a pill or capsule, dip the pill in maple syrup first. The pill will slide down the patient's throat more easily this way.

Dianne Charron, RN, BSN

That's the breaks

Here's an easy way to break a scored pill in half. Just insert a sterile needle into the groove. The pill will break apart cleanly.

Barbara Birkenberger, RN

Scalped pills

Keep a disposable scalpel on your medication cart to cut pills in half. Just remember to clean the scalpel with a povidone-iodine or alcohol swab before and after each use.

Carol Brower, RN

Powdered pill

When you need to crush pills for a patient who can't swallow them, try using a hemostat instead of a mortar and pestle. Leave the pills in their plastic unit-dose package and squeeze them with the hemostat. This method is easy, eliminates cleanup, and ensures that the patient receives the full dose.

Connie Norheim, RN

Fast way to crush medication

I use a pestle to crush medication right in the packaging. This saves time because I don't have to use the mortar and don't have anything to clean—I can just throw away the packaging after I've removed the medication.

Derenda Whitefield, RN

Quick crush

I work primarily with geriatric patients, and I have to crush a lot of medications. I've found a quick, sanitary way to do that. I put the tablet in a paper cup and place an empty cup inside the first, on top of the tablet. Then I pound a pestle into the top cup. This easily crushes the tablet, and the pieces are neatly contained in one cup.

Jan M. Moroni, RN, BSN

Taking medication in one swallow

We dissolve certain drugs in a small amount of water to make them easier to swallow. (Of course, we check with the pharmacist before doing this to make sure the drug can be dissolved.) But some of the medication may adhere to the sides of a plastic cup. I discovered that this doesn't happen with waxed paper cups. So the patient receives the entire dose of medication in one swallow.

Mari-Ellen Barasch, RN, BSN

Quick dissolve

If you have to administer tablets or capsules through a nasogastric tube because no liquid replacements are available, remember that the medication will dissolve more rapidly and completely in *warm* water. And since less warm water is needed to dissolve the medication, a patient on fluid restriction won't get too much liquid.

Barbara A. Matheus, RN, BSN

Faster fizz

Potassium bicarbonate or potassium chloride tablets can take a long time to dissolve in cold water. To speed up the process, I put them in a small amount of lukewarm water and add the prescribed amount of cold water (or clear soda) once they've dissolved. This way, the tablets dissolve in a minute—saving time when I'm busy.

Sheryl Stone Clay, RN, BSN

In good measure

When you give patients liquid oral medications, suggest that they rinse out and save the plastic medicine cups. The cups will help them measure liquid medication accurately after they leave the hospital.

Jeri L. Hoover, RN

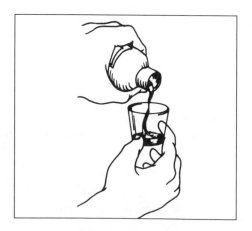

Handy storage for insulin bottles

We have a great way to store insulin bottles in our refrigerator. We keep them in small ice cube trays. That way, the bottles don't roll around or get lost. And because we can read the labels at a glance, we don't have to search for what we need.

Sharon Stratton, RN, BSN

Cutting suppositories the right way

If you need to cut a suppository in half, cut it lengthwise. Suppositories are tapered, so there's less of the drug at the tip. If you cut the suppository in half widthwise, the patient wouldn't get the right amount of medication.

However, check with the pharmacy before you cut the suppository—a lower strength may be available.

Pediatric nursing staff, Long Island College Hospital

Dosage markers

Elderly diabetic patients who give themselves insulin sometimes have trouble reading the unit markings on the syringe. To prevent a dosage error, use a marking pen or colored nail polish to mark the correct number of units on each syringe.

Ruth L. Nermal, RN

Twist-off cap off

If you're ever stuck with a hard-to-open pour-bottle of liquid medication, try wrapping any flat piece of rubber 1½ times around the cap. Rubber tourniquets are ideal. You'll find that the cap will unscrew with just a gentle twist.

Diane Puta, RN

Administration

Calculating with confidence

As a busy nursing supervisor, I taped a small list of dosage calculations to the back of my identification badge.

Now when I'm in a crunch, I have quick access to this information. I've taught my staff to do the same, which has saved time and boosted confidence in our unit.

Jacqueline Zabresky, RN, BA

Without a doubt

If a patient questions the color, shape, or number of pills you're about to give him, double-check your medication order before you give the pills. The patient may be right.

Emilie M. Tese, RN

Wrapped until ready

When administering medications, I leave them in their unit-dose blister packages until I get to the patient's bedside. Then I open one medication at a time, say its name out loud, and proceed with patient teaching. This helps prevent medication errors.

Marietta B. Mukiibi, RN

Sound regimen

Patients who take medications several times a day might benefit from this reminder system my husband uses. He's had glaucoma for several years and must use eyedrops six times a day. To help him stay on schedule, we bought an electronic kitchen timer that can be "triple set"—that is, set to ring at three different times. When it rings for the third time, we reset the timer for the next three medication times.

Helen Hibbs, RN

Full dose for infants

Getting an infant to take an entire dose of oral medication may be difficult. I dip the outer part of a nipple in a liquid the infant likes, then I insert the medication-filled syringe into the nipple. I can administer the medication as the infant sucks, and he gets the full dose.

Diane Lyness, BSN

Easy dose it

Babies and toddlers who've had surgery are frequently given antibiotics by mouth because their I.V. lines have been discontinued. We've found a way to give these liquid medications without spills and dribbles. We cut the tip off a disposable nipple, pour the medication into the tip, and let the child suck on it. The baby gets an accurate dose, and we save time.

Susan R. Potts, RN

Let's pretend

Trying to get a 2-year-old to take medicine can be a real battle. Before he has to take antibiotics or cough medicine, pretend to give some to a doll. After watching a "sick" dolly take the medicine, the child will happily take his dose.

Patricia Trefethen, RN

Hugging mommy

Here's a way to make preoperative injections less traumatic for young children, and for you, too. Have the child sit on his mother's lap and hug her while you're giving the injection. Hugging mommy gives the child a feeling of security and keeps his muscles relaxed while you're insert-ing the needle. If the child begins to fight back, his mother simply hugs him tighter. This is much nicer than having strangers hold the child while he's getting his injection.

Phyllis A. Smith, RN

Functional funnel

I use a funnel made from a plastic probe to give sublingual medications to comatose or intubated patients. I snip a corner off the end of the probe and insert it into the patient's mouth. Then I position it so the medication can be placed in the proper area. After administering the medication, I flush the probe with a

few drops of water to make sure he receives the full dose.

Gary Walters, RN, BSN

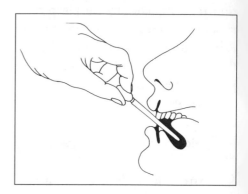

Sublingual access

Several of my geriatric patients take sublingual nitroglycerin. To make sure the tablet is properly placed, I gently lift the tongue with a tongue

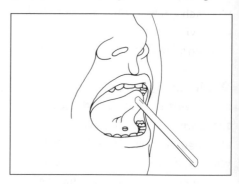

blade instead of my finger and put the pill in the sublingual area.

Connie Granada, RN, BSN

Squirt with a syringe

Sometimes you may have trouble administering nifedipine (Procardia) sublingually if a patient is particularly confused or lethargic. Instead of struggling to express the liquid directly from the capsule into his mouth, you can administer it with a tuberculin syringe. Here's how: First, break open the capsule and empty the contents into a medicine cup. Then, draw the liquid into a tuberculin syringe. Finally, administer it sublingually. (You don't use a needle, of course.) This method gives you more control, and it ensures that the patient will receive the full dose.

Mary E. Fassetta, RN, MS

Handy stopcock

You can give medications quickly to patients receiving feedings through small-bore Silastic tubes by attaching a 3-way stopcock to the tube. This allows you to give medications without disconnecting the tube, which could create a mess. It also provides easy access when you need to flush the tube.

Bonnie Alvey, RN

No clumps

To administer crushed pills through a feeding tube, follow this procedure. Make sure the pills are properly crushed. Put the powder in a 30-ml measuring cup and add 1 tablespoon of applesauce (after making sure the patient can have applesauce) and a little warm water. Stir well, then put the mixture in a syringe and administer through the tube. Flush with water.

The applesauce will suspend the powdered medication so it won't clump in the syringe or tube.

Debbie Hagerty, RN

Mix that won't clog tube

Administering a powder laxative like psyllium (Metamucil) through a feeding or gastrostomy tube can be difficult. Try mixing it first with juice. To make sure the solution won't clog the tube, flush immediately with water.

Linda Neal, RN

Lots of water—or a banana

Pills or capsules will sometimes linger in the esophagus, especially if a patient takes them while lying down and drinks only a small amount of water. This creates a significant risk of esophagitis.

I have two suggestions for avoiding this problem: First, have the patient stand, if possible, to take pills

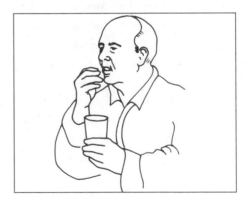

or capsules. And ask him to remain standing for about a minute and a half after taking the medication. Also, he should drink at least a cup of water.

The second suggestion is for patients who can't stand. Have them eat a few bits of a banana after taking a pill or capsule. The banana will coat the pill or capsule and help it pass smoothly through the esophagus.

Hans H. Neumann, MD

Wiggle while you work

Before I give a patient an I.M. injection, I ask him to take a deep breath and to wiggle his toes. This is a good distractor—and a good icebreaker.

Doreen Eyre-Baker, RN

Keeping tabs on injection sites

I work on a busy surgical unit and administer I.M. pain medications to postoperative patients. To help us rotate each patient's injection sites, we use the side rails of the bed as reminders. If the last injection was given on the patient's left side, we put a piece of adhesive tape on the left side rail of his bed; if the injection was given on the right side, we put the tape on the right side rail. We tab the tape so it can be easily removed and reapplied on the opposite side rail after the next injection.

Rachel Raguso, RN, BSN

Easing the pain of a potassium I.V.

Potassium I.V. solutions irritate a patient's vein. To ease the discomfort, I gently apply an ice pack at the infusion site. Also, I periodically clamp off the I.V., take down the container, and quickly invert it twice

so the potassium doesn't settle at the bottom.

Doris A. Millam, RN, CRNI, MS

Easy application

One of our patients recently had a deep, sacral pressure ulcer. The doctor ordered an ointment to be instilled directly into the ulcer. But trying to get the ointment from the jar to the ulcer with a cotton swab proved awkward.

To solve this problem, we asked the pharmacist to put the ointment in a tube. Then, to apply the ointment, we put a new applicator tip from a hemorrhoidal ointment preparation on the tube. The ointment went neatly into the ulcer, with little waste.

Maria Schmitt, RN

Band it

Instead of using tape to secure a topical application of nitroglycerin (Nitrol) on a patient's arm, use a stretch terrycloth wristband. The patient won't have to remove and put on more sticky, irritating tape each time he needs another application.

Ruth Petkus, RN

Documentation

Facts at your fingertips

In our emergency department (ED), we keep a "pertinent facts" rotary card file by the phone. The file lists childhood communicable diseases and immunization schedules, tetanus booster requirements, acetaminophen (Tylenol) doses, and community agencies ED personnel might need to know, such as battered-women's shelters. Arranged alphabetically, the resource list often comes in handy.

Jan Widman, RN

Medication card

A nurse on the dialysis unit where I work designed a wallet-sized medication card for patients to carry. The front of the card gives information in the event of an emergency. It looks like this:

Name _____
Address _____
City _____
Phone _____
Dialysis mode
☐ Hemo   ☐ IPO   ☐ CAPD
Access _____
Days ☐ M-W-F   ☐ T-Th-Sat   ☐ __
MD _____
Blood type_____
☐ PRCS   ☐ WPRC
Allergies_____
_____
Emergency contact_____
_____
Relation _____
Phone _____

NOTE: Patient may have received heparin recently.

The reverse side of the card is headed "MEDICATIONS" and has blank lines for the names of the patient's medications. We update each patient's list whenever his medication is changed, during his primary nurse's monthly review, and upon his discharge from the hospital.

Patients and their families appreciate the medication cards because the cards help them remember what medications the patient is taking. Nurses like them because they speed admission procedures. And emergency personnel appreciate knowing the patient's history and course of treatment.

Jeanette K. Chambers, RN, CS, MS

Medication information

Here's a way to keep track of medications administered on a unit: Post a sheet of paper on the door of the narcotics cabinet. As each narcotic (sedative, pain reliever, or whatever) is administered, record on the sheet the patient's name, room number, medication, and time it was administered. The sheet provides (1) a quick reference to indicate when a patient received his last medication, (2) a vital information list for the shift report, and (3) a checklist for the narcotic count at the end of each shift.

A.E. Siminski, RN

Double check on drugs

To prevent drug interactions, you need to know what medications a patient is taking when he's admitted to the hospital and where those medications are being kept during his hospitalization. Recording this information on the back of the patient's Kardex works well. The information is right at your fingertips whenever it's needed.

Doris Sedberry, LVN

Patch and paste pointers

When I apply nitroglycerin to a patient, I write the patient's blood pressure on the patch or paste paper, in addition to the date and time. I also indicate on the medication administration record where I've placed the patch or paste. This way, other nurses can easily find it.

Theresa M. Dando, RN, BSN

10 SAFETY

Double-checking a chart
When you're checking a patient's order sheet, always make sure the orders were written for the intended patient. Occasionally an order sheet may be stamped with one patient's ID plate but inadvertently placed in another patient's chart. By double-checking, you'll avoid potential mistakes.

Edwina A. McConnell, RN, PhD

Allergy alert
In our postanesthesia care unit, we have standing orders to administer morphine sulfate or meperidine I.V. to patients who need pain relief. There may be a patient who's allergic to one of these drugs, so we tape a written warning to the I.V. pole, where it's easily seen.

Marci Smith, RN, BS

Taped ties
For the patient who has a tracheostomy tube, there is a constant danger of aspirating a loose thread from the frayed ends of the ties. But eliminating this danger is simple: Just cover the ends of the ties with nylon tape. To further ensure the patient's safety (and comfort), knot the tie at the side rather than the back of his neck, so it won't cause irritation when he lies on his back.

Diana Contine, RN

Shock stopper
To protect patients with temporary pacemakers from electric shock, cover the pacemaker's unconnected wires with rubber tops from used Tubex syringes. The rubber tops ground the wires and can easily be removed when the wires are needed.

Bernie Stremikis, RN, BSN

Sterile supplies
Remember that everyday supplies like bandage scissors, hemostats, and penlights can cause cross-contamination if you don't keep them clean. I soak mine in a 50% bleach solution for 1 to 2 hours to sterilize them. And I use alcohol wipes to clean the bell and diaphragm of my stethoscope between patients.

Linnette Angell-Drouin, SN

Mouth guard magic

If a comatose patient with cerebral hemorrhage continually grinds his teeth and bites his lower lip, prevent further damage by using a football mouth guard. Soften it in warm water, and fit it over his lower teeth. Next, thread trach tape through the first hole of the guard's 6" helmet strap. Finally, run one tape end over each ear and tie the ends behind the patient's head—loosely enough to be comfortable, but tightly enough to hold the guard in place if he coughs.

You can buy the guard at most sporting goods stores.

Tina Sykes, LPN

Evac-pack

When we have tornado warnings, we have to evacuate patients from our alcoholism rehabilitation unit to an underground tunnel. Sometimes we have to stay in the tunnel for as long as an hour or more, and the patients get restless.

To alleviate their boredom and to be prepared in case of an emergency, we've prepared a "tornado pack." These items—stored in a wash basin and enclosed in a plastic bag—are included in our pack:
• adhesive bandages
• alcohol swabs
• ammonia ampuls
• battery-powered radio
• blood pressure cuff
• emesis basin

• flashlight
• hard candy
• Kardex with patient census
• name bands
• pens
• plastic cups
• playing cards
• prepackaged towelettes
• safety pins
• stethoscope
• tissues
• tongue blades.

The pack is always ready to move whenever we are.

Terry Clayburn, RN
Rita Biggs, LPN

Wrist watching

When a patient has I.V.s infusing in both wrists, what do you do with his wrist ID band? If the I.V. in the wrist with the ID band infiltrates, the wrist might swell, making the band too tight and impairing circulation.

To prevent this, make a slit in one end of the wristband before you put it on the patient. Put a rubber band through the slit, pull the two loop ends of the rubber band into the metal clasp, and close the clasp. Now you have a stretch wristband that will "grow" if necessary.

Sally Sumner, RN

Preventing mistaken identity

In our mental health unit, patients aren't required to wear armbands with their names on them—which presents a problem for float nurses who pass out medications. We solved this by taking a photo of each patient, labeling it with his name, and placing it in his medication profile. Now a float nurse can look up the patient's picture for easy identification, saving time and preventing medication errors.

D. Fisk, RN

Finding yourself

As you go from one patient's room to another, you can easily forget which room you're in if the number's not posted inside. This could cause a delay if you had to call a code or call for help.

To solve this problem, mark each room's telephone (or some other central object) with the room number on fluorescent tape. You can also use a fluorescent marker or crayon to write the number on white paper, then tape it to the phone.

Whichever way you choose, the room number will be clearly visible—even in the dark.

Margaret Beckert, RN

Reducing falls: Blue alert

We place a blue ID bracelet on a disoriented or unsteady patient. Because the bracelet alerts staff that the patient needs assistance when he's mobile, it helps reduce the risk of falls.

Tammy Clark, LPN

Yellow alert

In our hospital, we give patients who are at risk for falling mustard-yellow gowns to wear. This easy identification helps staff prevent a lot of falls.

Carolyn P. Cave, RN

Wheelchair safety

To stress wheelchair safety and make it enjoyable, nurses at Memorial Hospital of Southern Oklahoma, Ardmore, offer a class in wheelchair safety and award a "driver's license" to employees and volunteers who complete the class.

Personnel assigned to transporting patients in wheelchairs, attend a 1½-hr class where they learn how to ascend and descend a ramp with an occupied wheelchair, how to use footrests, how to comfortably secure a helpless patient in a wheelchair, and more. After successfully completing the class, participants receive a driver's license.

The director of inservice education at the hospital says she plans to put the "rules of the halls" on the back of the licenses. For now, though, personnel are proud of their driver's licenses—and their proven skill in transporting patients.

Lenna Lee Davidson, RN, MPH

Restraining patients without restraints

Instead of using wrist restraints to keep a confused or combative patient from hurting his hands or pulling at his I.V. tubes, drains, or dressings, we put a soft washcloth in each hand, then wrap the fists closed with gauze. For quick access to the patient's hands, we can just cut away the gauze.

Sandra McCarver, RN, CCRN

"Seat belt" safety

When I must restrain a patient, I tell him to think of the restraint as a seat belt. He won't be as upset if he knows the restraint is for his own safety.

Brenda Callihan, RN

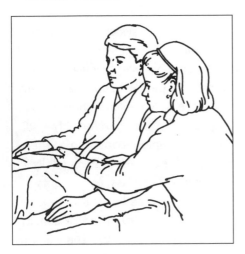

Extending side rails

If side rails don't go the length of the bed, you can easily extend them. Simply place a footboard on either side of the bed where the rails end. The patient won't be able to throw his legs over the edge of the bed, so he won't be in danger of falling. And you might not have to restrain him.

Valerie Davis, LPN

Protective sleeve for fragile skin

Here's an inexpensive way to protect an elderly patient's fragile skin:

Cut a piece of orthopedic stockinette that's long enough to cover the patient's arm from the hand to the elbow. Slip the stockinette over his arm, then cut a small hole to slide his thumb through (this will hold the stockinette in place).

Now if he bumps his arm, his skin will be less likely to tear. Just remember to remove the stockinette as needed for skin care and assessment.

Karen Seifert, RN

On guard

At the nursing home where I work, we place shin guards over our patient's arms and legs to minimize skin tears. The cloth-covered foam guards provide a protective barrier against hard surfaces. Also, the pads help reduce hypothermia by keeping the extremities warm.

Maxine Chisholm, MSN, GNP

Safe stairs for the elderly

Falling is always a risk for an elderly person, especially if he lives in a house with lots of stairs. Here are a few tips that family members can use to help make his home safer:

• Paint the first and last steps on the stairs using a color that's different from the room. The paint will make the steps easier to see.

• If the stairs have a banister, place a knob on the banister at the first and last steps to serve as a signal.
• Outside stairs can become slick when wet. Before painting the steps, add sand to the paint. When the paint dries, you'll have a rough surface that should prevent slipping.

Arlene Orhon Jech, RN

Eye openers

For my elderly home health care patients who can't see the small numbers on their stoves and microwaves, I put brightly colored stickers above the numbers they use most. This way they can more easily recognize the numbers and temperatures, preventing them from burning themselves and starting fires.

Debbie Sanders, RN

Catheter bag hang-up

Keeping your hands free can be difficult when helping a patient with an I.V. line and indwelling urinary catheter to walk. Here's a way to solve the problem:

Tape two wooden tongue blades together, then use masking tape to secure them low on the I.V. pole.

Now you have a notch to hang the catheter bag on, leaving your hands free to grasp the patient's transfer belt and prevent him from falling.

Alicia Vano Truttmann, LPN, SN, EMT

It's a wrap

If you've ever tried to help your patients out of a bathtub, you know they can be hard to handle once they're wet. To gain control, place a towel under each of the patient's arms and hold the ends near his shoulders. If you need more control, grasp the towel closer to the patient's body; if you want the towel looser, just allow a little slack.

Fatima Bayati, RN

Pad-a-tub

To keep our patients from slipping and falling in the bathtub, we put a convoluted foam mattress in the bottom of the tub. The mattress gives the patients a sure footing when they get into and out of the tub. It also makes the tub more comfortable to sit in. After a patient's bath, we discard the mattress or squeeze the water out of it and let it dry.

Joyce Kron, RN

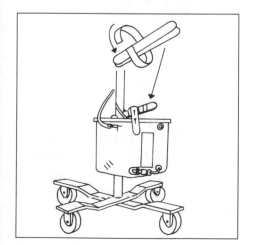

Shock-absorbing sock

Some of my patients who take pred-nisone develop bruises on their arms when they do housework or yard work. So I suggest they wear white sport socks (with the feet cut off) on their arms. The socks cushion any impact and are easily hidden under long-sleeved shirts and blouses.

Techia McGrath, RN

Slippers with stick

If the soles of a patient's slippers are smooth, I put masking tape on them. The tape provides traction and is an inexpensive way to help prevent falls.

Teresa D. Leese, LPN

Slipper holder

Do your patients' slippers seem to play hide-and-seek under their beds? Retrieving these slippers is not only a nuisance for you, but also a danger for patients, especially the elderly and those with balance problems or limited vision.

Make a slipper holder. All you need is a piece of heavy-duty cloth or canvas, about 16" wide x 10" long. Stitch two pockets—about 6" x 8" long—to the front of the cloth. Attach strings to the upper corners so the holder can be tied to the side rail or frame of the bed.

Becky Schroeder, RN

A pedigreed clamp

I teach my patients who have indwelling central venous catheters to use bulldog clamps instead of plastic or padded Kelly clamps, which are not only awkward but may damage the catheter. The bull-dog clamps are small, lightweight, inexpensive, easy to handle, and don't need to be padded. And they fit easily on neck chains or bracelets so patients can keep them handy at all times.

Linda Barr, RN, CCN

A lid latch

Do you find that a commode lid often slams shut just as you lower a patient onto the seat? Not only is this frustrating for you, but it's also dangerous to the patient. Here's a way to keep the lid raised:

Get a Velcro book latch (usually used to hold large chart pages open). The book latch has 2 parts: a long tab and a circle. Both parts have adhesive backs that stick to almost any surface.

Attach the adhesive side of the long tab to the underside of the commode lid. Then attach the adhe-sive side of the circle to the front of the commode frame with one end of the tab hanging down. (The tab's Velcro side should face backward.)

Before you help a patient onto the commode, lift the lid. Bring the tab up over the lid and secure it to the circle on the lid. The lid will remain raised until you undo the latch.

Ruth C. Flowe, LPN

A glass assignment

A patient's eyeglasses can easily be knocked off his bedside table and broken. To prevent such an accident, I tape a plastic emesis basin to the table and write the word "glasses" on the tape (so the basin won't be removed). The patient can put his glasses in the basin, where they're less likely to slide off the table and break.

Laurie Roper, LPN

Denture dots

Has the "lost denture epidemic" struck the hospital where you work? You know the causes: A patient removes his dentures and puts them on his meal tray or beside his pillow instead of in his denture cup. Later, when the tray is taken away or the bed is changed, the dentures are inadvertently thrown out or they fall on the floor and break.

We've halted this epidemic by placing a self-adhesive red dot on the headboard of the bed of each patient who wears dentures. We put another red dot on the patient's Kardex. The dots remind staff to look carefully for stray dentures on meal trays before removing them, among linens when changing beds, and in tissues and cups when straightening the bedside tables.

When the patient leaves the hospital, we remove the red dot from the bed and the Kardex.

Our red dot prevention program has saved our hospital a lot of money—no more lawsuits against the hospital for broken or lost dentures, no more staff time spent looking for lost dentures. And it's saved our patients the inconvenience of being without their dentures.

Barbara S. Vosburgh, Patient Relations Services

Blowing the whistle

A police whistle is an excellent home health care safety device for an elderly person or someone who uses a wheelchair. If the person falls, he can blow the whistle to summon help. Police whistles require little breath to make a loud sound and can be worn around the neck for easy access.

Terrilynn M. Quillen, RN

Signal for help

A patient who's at high risk for falling and injuring himself may have trouble using a call bell. Here's how I solve the problem:

I place a pancake-type call bell (an oval-shaped bell that's extremely sensitive to any pressure or touch) between his gown and the front of his vest restraint. If the patient doesn't have a vest restraint, I fasten the pancake bell to his gown with tape.

The bell is activated when the patient becomes restless or tries to remove the vest restraint. So I'm sure to be alerted if he needs help or if he's about to fall out of bed.

Krystyna Paech, RN,C

Emergency necklace

A patient who has a fractured mandible that's wired and banded should always keep wire cutters nearby in case of an emergency. But remembering to carry the wire cutters with him can be a problem. That's why we make a "necklace" from tracheostomy tape and put the wire cutters on the tape. The patient wears the necklace wherever he goes (except to bed, when he leaves it on his bedside table) so the wire cutters are always handy in an emergency.

Vicki Cornish, RN, BSN

Alarm alert for the elderly

Here's a safety tip for elderly patients who use a walker, especially those who live alone in apartment buildings: Tie a wall-mount fire alarm onto the walker, with the testing button facing the patient. Alert his neighbors that you're doing this. Then if the patient falls, he can press the button and they'll come to his aid.

Margaret E. Ivester, RN

Calling for help

Before his discharge, I encourage a new tracheotomy or laryngectomy patient—or a family member—to record an emergency message on a cassette tape. The message should clearly state the patient's name, address, telephone number, and type of airway, and that he requires emergency assistance immediately. I encourage him to keep the cassette in a tape recorder by the phone. If he needs help, he has only to dial the phone number, push the play button, and place the handset next to the recorder's speaker.

Colleen A. Carey, RN, BSN

Bright idea

A patient with impaired vision who has an emergency call-cord in his apartment will be able to see the cord much better if he ties a fluorescent table-tennis ball to the end of it.

Lynda R. Dunlop, RN, BSN

Staff safety

Garbage bags as protective gowns

We care for many patients who have gastrointestinal bleeding or AIDS. But we don't think the flimsy disposable gowns we wear protect us from spraying blood. So we've come up with a solution:

We cut holes for our heads and arms in large, clear plastic garbage bags. We keep a supply of these handy and wear them whenever we do a procedure. Because the garbage bags are clear, patients can still see our uniforms and name tags.

Linda Fish, RN, BSN, MA

Isolation protection

To ease the fear often associated with caring for patients in isolation, including patients with AIDS, our staff keeps a pocket mask on the cart outside each isolated patient's room. We also keep a mask in each team conference center and on each crash cart. Our staff-development department has taught us the proper way to use the masks to administer cardiopulmonary resuscitation.

Debbie Bornholdt, RN, BSN

Cover-up for cuts

To protect small cuts on your hands from infection and irritation, cover the cuts with occlusive I.V. dressings. The dressings are flexible, and they'll stay in place when you wash your hands.

Jennie Ruley, RN

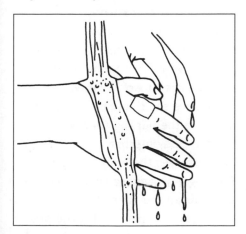

Cot for cover

Here's how I keep the bell of my stethoscope clean and free of germs: I cover the bell with a finger cot. The cot stretches easily, fits snugly, and saves me from frequently washing the bell with alcohol.

Linda J.H. Baker, RN

Posting an important protocol

Every health care worker should know what to do after a needle stick or other exposure to blood and body fluids. We keep a laminated copy of our hospital's protocol—and the supplies needed to treat an exposure—in the unit's clean utility room. Because staff members have quick access to the step-by-step instructions, they're reassured that they're correctly following the procedure.

Joan Neer LaComb, RN

Sharps safety

When I start an I.V. infusion or perform a fingerstick on a patient, I place a clean emesis basin at my side. The basin provides a safe place for needles, lancets, and I.V. catheter stylets until I can walk across the room to put the items in the sharps container.

Cynthia Mik, RN, CDE

Removing a lancet safely

After testing a diabetic patient's

blood glucose level, I use my hemostat to remove the lancet from the
plunger. I can firmly grasp the lancet
with the hemostat, which lessens
the chance that I'll accidentally
puncture my skin.

Diane Rakestraw, RN

Mobile blood samples

As a home health care nurse, I often
draw and transport blood for analysis. To protect myself from contact
with a patient's blood, here's what I
do:

After filling and capping the vial, I
hold it in one gloved hand. Then I
pull the glove off and over the vial
with the other hand. The vial will fit

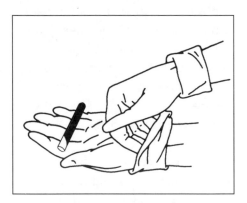

into one of the fingers of the glove.
If the blood must be kept cold, I fill
the glove with ice. I tie the open
end of the glove with the thumb to
form a waterproof container.

Aileen Walters, RN

Recycling plastic bottles

As in most operating rooms, we use
many plastic liter bottles of normal
saline solution and sterile water. We
save empty bottles, then drain the
contents of indwelling urinary
catheter bags and other drains into
them. After tightly capping the lid,
we place the entire bottle into a
hazardous waste trash bag.

Now we no longer have to carry
open containers of bodily fluids
through the operating room to the
utility room, plus we're doing our
part in the recycling effort by using
one container instead of two.

Arline M. Brice, RN
Jane Arrendell, RN

Traction protection

Bars protruding from a traction
setup are not only a nuisance, but
also dangerous to staff and visitors.
Make them injury-proof by placing
soft sponge rubber balls on the protruding ends. The balls cushion any
contact with the sharp ends. And,
since you use bright red balls, people see them from a distance *before*
coming in contact with the bars.

Della Anderson, RN

Check out the moves

When a staff member recovers
from a sprain or strain (frequently
suffered while lifting a heavy patient)
and returns to work, we want to
make sure she doesn't hurt herself
again. So the nursing supervisor
does a "body mechanics review."
She observes the employee performing a procedure similar to one
that caused the injury. If the
employee isn't performing the pro-

cedure according to correct body mechanics, the supervisor refers her to the physical therapy department for instructions in body mechanics. Staffers appreciate this review and so does hospital administration—because it helps reduce the number of repeat injuries and time lost from work.

Joanne Beden, RN

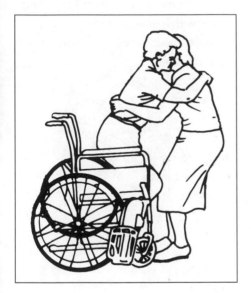

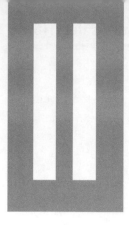

COST AND TIMESAVER TIPS

Equipment

Easy tubing change

When you replace the rubber tubing on a stethoscope, put a small amount of liquid soap on the metal section. That will help you slide the tubing on more easily and the tubing will stay put when the soap dries. Oils or jellies remain slippery.

Try this when you replace the bulb on a blood pressure cuff, too.

Bob Anderson, RN

Ice packs: Banding together

Try using sweatbands to keep an ice pack in place. They're often effective for holding packs in awkward positions, such as on the patient's jaw after a tooth extraction. They're washable and inexpensive.

Charlotte Wood, MSN

Handy spot for tonsil suction catheter

I've had trouble finding a convenient place for a tonsil suction catheter when I wasn't using it. Here's my solution: I cut a long piece of tape

and wind it most of the way around the suction canister. Then I tape the package that the catheter came in to the canister. This way, I can insert

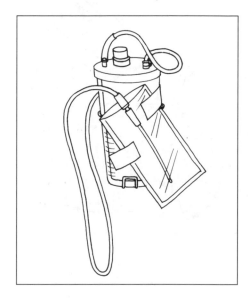

the catheter into the package after each use and avoid contamination. The package holds the catheter in place and keeps it from falling on the floor.

Lori Brown, RN

Tube tidiness

If your patient needs frequent suctioning, secure a 10-ml syringe barrel to the suction canister so that you can place the end of the tubing in the barrel. Make sure the canister is positioned at waist level or higher. With this setup, you always have a clean place for the suction tubing.

Polly Gerber Zimmermann, RN, CEN, BSN, MBA

Position a mattress with powder

Here's a simple way to slide a convoluted foam mattress back into position:

Pull the sheets out from both sides of the bed and sprinkle powder between the top of the regular mattress and the bottom of the convoluted mattress. Rub the powder as far under that mattress as you can. Now it will easily slide back into position.

If a sheet is over the regular mattress, just push it to the center of the bed before applying the powder.

Dot Wiegand, RN

Light cord with a ring

We tie the overhead light cord to the side rail of the patient's bed. Sometimes, though, we can't untie the knot we've made, so we have to cut the cord before moving the bed. That leaves an ugly, frayed cord that's too short to use.

We solved this problem by tying the end of a cord to a plastic toddler play ring—the kind with an opening in it. We make sure there's enough slack in the cord for lowering the side rail. Then we simply

snap the ring over the side rail.

When we have to move the bed, we can easily take the ring off the side rail. Plus, the patient can quickly locate the light cord with the ring.

Lynn Martin, RN, EMT-P

A flip tip

Each time a patient's bed linens are completely changed, or at least twice a week, the mattress also should be flipped. Flipping the mattress preserves its life and makes for greater patient comfort.

Charles Koltz, RN

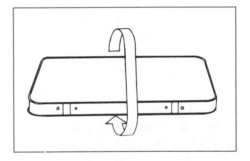

Supplies

Postmortem pack

To prevent losing hospital linens to mortuaries when transferring a deceased patient, I designed a low-cost "postmortem pack" for my facility. Each pack contains a disposable isolation gown and two 48" x 48" sterile wrappers. We dress the deceased patient in the gown and then place both wrappers under the body, reaching from shoulders to knees. We use the wrappers to lift the body onto the morgue cart and then onto the funeral home stretcher. These cost-effective wrappers support up to 300 pounds.

Margaret P. Taylor, RN

Preparing for morning care

When I work the 3-to-11 shift, the other nursing assistants and I restock a cart with sheets, blankets, lift pads, pillowcases, gowns, towels, washcloths, and personal hygiene items. Then we place it midway down the hall against the wall. This way, nursing staff members don't have to go back and forth to the clean utility room for those items during morning patient care.

Pamela Curran, NA

Early morning setup

When I'm on the 11-to-7 shift at our long-term care facility, I try to do some advance work for the 7-to-3 nurses, who have the busier shift. One thing I do is set up a tray with all the supplies they'll need for certain treatments, tube feedings, and special procedures that day. Of course, I leave these items in their sterile containers.

Teresa D. Liesi, LPN

Cost containment for your unit

Like many staff nurses, you may not know the cost of items used in patient care. Yet cost containment is important at every hospital. Here's

what you can do to become more aware of costs: Ask central supply to put a price tag on every item you keep in the central service cart. This may prompt you to choose less-expensive alternatives. For example, a 4" x 4" gauze pad may cost less and do the job as well as a more expensive dressing.

You might want to have a contest and give a reward for the most cost-effective nurse. If you try this, you may end up saving money for your unit.

Edwina A. McConnell, RN, PhD

Saving 4" x 4" gauze pads

When my 3-month-old daughter had to wear a hip brace, I taped 4" x 4" gauze pads to the sides of the brace to protect her skin. Because she had frequent bowel movements, I had to change the gauze pads often—too often, since the gauze and tape were expensive.

Then I decided to try using thin sanitary pads, cut to size, instead. I found the pads cheaper to use than gauze, and since they have an adhesive backing, I didn't have to buy adhesive tape anymore, either.

Maisie Hubbard, RN, MSN

Cost-cutting care

When my grandfather needed a new colostomy irrigation bag, I went shopping for it at the local drugstore. I found an inexpensive alternative: a douche bag. The douche bag does the job as well as a colostomy irrigation bag, but it's sturdier and costs about one third less.

Linda Harrish, LPN

Irrigating? Think small.

When a patient has a small fistula or wound that needs to be irrigated frequently, don't use a big 1,000-ml bottle of normal saline solution. It just clutters the patient's bedside table, and later, the unused solution will have to be discarded.

Use 5-ml vials of normal saline solution instead. A few vials are usually sufficient for each irrigation.

Mary E. Anderson, RN, MSN

A pointer on catheterization

When learning how to insert a urinary catheter into a female patient, a student sometimes contaminates several catheters just trying to locate the meatus. To cut down on catheter waste, I have the student open a package of sterile cotton-tipped applicators onto the sterile field. Then she puts on her gloves, picks up an applicator, and points to where she intends to insert the catheter. If she needs help, I can use another applicator to show her where the catheter should be positioned.

Using applicators saves the time and expense of repeated catheterizations. But most of all, it saves your patient the embarrassment and discomfort of a prolonged catheter insertion.

Connie Norehim, RN, BSN, MSEd

Squeeze 'n' freeze

You can make your own ice pack by sealing a wet sponge in a plastic bag and freezing it. The size of the sponge can vary, depending on the injury site. The sponges contain no chemicals, so they can be applied near the eye. And they're reusable.

Arlene Evans, RN

Cold pack covers

Paper booties from the operating room make great covers for gel-filled cold packs. They slide easily over the packs, and I've found that they're thicker and more absorbent than the commercially manufactured "sleeves" we had been using. Plus, they're more hygienic than a folded washcloth secured with tape, another option we had explored.

Terrilynn M. Quillen, RN

Rubbery remedy

Here's what I do to create a rubber-tipped hemostat: I save the red, rubber needle covers from empty prefilled opioid syringes. When I need a rubber-tipped hemostat, I cut a cover in half and place the halves over the tips of my hemostat. I change the halves if they become contaminated.

Ruth A. Slade, RN

No more torn tapes

A paper measuring tape can tear easily when you're using it frequently to measure limbs or abdominal girth. So I cover both sides of the measuring tape with paper tape. The paper tape is thin enough to let you see the numbers on the measuring tape—and sturdy enough to prevent the measuring tape from tearing.

Michaele Nesbitt-Johnson, RN

Exposed but not disposed

X-ray film can have a diverse after-life—after it's been exposed, that is. I use it as a notebook divider for patient profiles, narcotic books, and charts. I also write notes on it with a grease pencil. Later, I erase it with a clean gauze pad or cloth and use the film over again.

Jeri L. Hoover, Lt., NC, USN

Fresh approach

When one of my patients was both-ered by the odor in her room and I couldn't find a room deodorizer, I discovered an easy substitute. While trying to find the source of the odor, I moistened some paper tow-els with mouthwash and placed them in different spots around the room. The result—a clean, fresh smell.

Shirley Greuel, LPN

Peppermint-scented air

Sometimes you can't control the odor from a patient's infected wound or gastrointestinal bleeding. For an easy air freshener, try adding peppermint oil to a few cotton balls. Put the balls in paper medicine

cups and place them around the patient's room.

Also, before emptying a colosto-my bag, you can place a few drops of the peppermint oil in the bottom of the container you're using. Be sure to wash your hands after using the oil, because it's irritating to mucous membranes.

Christine Ozorio, RN, BSN

Recycling plastic bags

I've found a number of ways to reuse the large, flat, plastic bags that hold disposable underpads.

I use them to hold a patient's dirty linen or his personal items or to carry his toiletries to and from the shower. They're also good for weighing a pediatric patient's wet diaper.

Adrienne Ackley, LPN

Plastic bags for dirty laundry

Here's a recycling tip: Save the plas-tic bags covering new disposable bedpans and tuck them into the patient's drawer. His family can use them as laundry bags for his dirty clothing.

Mary H. Covell, RN,C, BS

Slipping personal items in a pocket

In a busy emergency department, keeping track of a patient's personal belongings can be difficult. So I tape a paper slipper to the head of the patient's bed. He can drop his eyeglasses or other small items in this paper "pocket" and they won't be misplaced. Or substitute a sealed envelope with one of its ends cut off.

Micky Antoniazzi, RN, EMT

Securing an NG tube

Here's an inexpensive way to secure a nasogastric (NG) tube to a patient's nose:

First, swab his nose with liquid adhesive to help the dressing adhere. Then use a Coverlet dressing to secure the tube. Place the wide end of the dressing over the bridge of the patient's nose and wrap the smaller end around the tube. The dressing won't irritate his nose and is less expensive than a box of regular nasal tube fasteners.

Patricia Bieniek, RNx

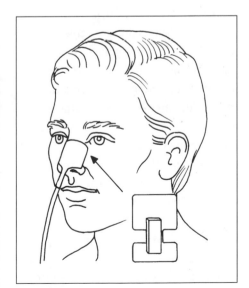

Traveling tissues

Because of his discomfort and trepidation, your postoperative patient

might forget to take tissues along when he starts walking again. To make sure the tissues go with him, put some in a plastic bag and pin the bag to his gown.

Kim Heiferman, RN

Smart totes

Our hospital's volunteer department provides handmade cotton tote bags for patients who must carry urinary or wound drainage containers in public. The sturdy bags hold the drainage containers discreetly, causing the patient far less embarrassment.

Jean Jackson, RN

Strong attachment

Try fastening Montgomery straps with Velcro instead of twill tape. Here's how: Attach a section of Velcro to each of four pieces of 2" to 3"-wide cloth tape. Position the tape on the dressing and close the Velcro.

The Velcro works well over areas

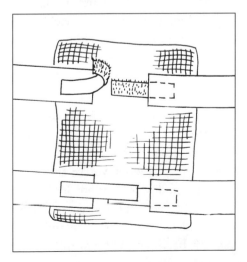

of copious drainage because it stays drier than twill tape. Also, it's not as bulky, opens and closes more easily, and holds the dressing in place just as well.

Kathy Ziembo, LPN

Catheter leg strap: Attractive alternative

Many female patients who need indwelling urinary catheters are bothered by the bulkiness and unsightliness of the anchoring leg strap. I suggest that they buy an inexpensive garter, then attach a loop of Velcro to hold the catheter in place. The result is far less unsightly, plus the homemade strap can cost less.

Terrilynn Quillen, RN

Clipping coupons

I work in a doctor's office. To help bring down the cost of medications and other health care items, we clip coupons from the newspaper and give them to our patients. These coupons are for discounts on new prescriptions at local pharmacies and for nonprescription items such as vitamins or eye care products.

Robbin McNamara, RN, BSN

Moving a mattress without a hassle

A convoluted foam mattress can be difficult to pull when you're transferring a bedridden patient from one bed to another. So I fold a bath blanket or sheet lengthwise and place it between the foam mattress

and the regular mattress. Then I can easily transfer the patient and foam mattress without worrying about tearing it.

Christine Ozorio, RN, BSN

Time

One-step chart removal

We have fire drills periodically to keep us prepared for an emergency. Getting the patients off the unit safely is our first priority, of course. But we also have to remove their charts. To do this easily, we use a sturdy laundry bag. We can remove the charts from the unit in one trip, and they'll all be together so we won't have to search for them later.

Lee DeKrey, RN,C, BSN

Hooray for the flags

With a little imagination, the "flags" on charts for stat orders can be used in many different ways. For instance, use them for evacuation drills. Put one—gray side out—on the outside door frame of the resident's room. During a drill, after making sure the room is empty, switch the stat flag to the red side.

Sean Damien, RN

Helpful hints: Easy as A to Z

I keep a pocket-sized address book with me and use it to jot down any helpful information—such as new drugs or doctors' names and specialties. Because my entries are in alphabetical order, I can quickly find what I'm looking for.

Mona Jacob, RN

Not carting disaster

Crash carts are necessary equipment in every hospital, of course. But because they're used less often than other equipment, our staff members weren't always able to locate the items in the cart quickly in an emergency. And sometimes certain items were missing from the cart.

To solve this problem, we took pictures of the inside of each fully stocked drawer. Then we pasted each picture and a list of that drawer's contents on separate pages in a loose-leaf binder. We laminated the pages for durability.

To ensure that the cart stays fully equipped, we banded each drawer so the band breaks if the drawer is opened.

We urge all staff members, and especially new employees, to study the loose-leaf binder periodically. Consequently, they're more familiar with the cart's contents and can function better in an emergency.

Banding the drawers assures that we'll be able to find all the necessary equipment when we need it.

Chris Chytraus, RN, BSN, CCRN

Cool tool

Every second counts during a code, so don't waste precious time look-ing for the proper size endotracheal tube. Have the linen department sew an expandable tube holder (similar to a silverware holder) out of muslin. Make a pocket for each tube and mark the tube size in large numbers on each pocket. Fasten a tie string on each end so you can roll the tube holder into a compact bundle and tie it, ready to use for the next code.

Chris McSharry, RN

Crash cart convenience

After working in the intensive care unit and recovery room for many years, I finally found a way to store endotracheal equipment on the crash cart neatly and conveniently.

First, I measured the depth, width, and length of the crash cart drawer and bought a flat piece of upholstery foam cut to that size. Then I laid all the endotracheal equipment (blades, handles, extra bulbs and batteries, forceps, and so on) on the foam and traced their outlines with a felt-tipped pen.

Next, I removed the equipment and, using my tracings as a guide, cut out their shapes in the foam with a scalpel blade, leaving a thin layer of uncut foam at the bottom of each shape. When finished, I placed the foam in the crash cart drawer and put the equipment in the cutout "pockets."

Now the equipment is easily visible and accessible, so I save time finding what I need during an emergency. And I can see immediately what's missing when I check the cart.

Susanne T. Smith, RN, BSN

Kits, carts, and emergency care #1

I work in a newborn nursery, but I'm frequently called to the delivery room or emergency department (ED) to give emergency care to a newborn in distress. Taking the crash cart along with me is difficult, time-consuming, and frequently unnecessary since I usually don't need all the supplies on it.

To save time and effort, I made a newborn emergency kit—a fishing tackle box stocked with the drugs and supplies I usually use in emergencies. Now when I get a call from the delivery room or ED, I just grab the emergency kit, and off I go.

The kit has worked so well that other nurses in the hospital have adapted it for diabetic patients: They stock a tackle box with supplies needed for hypoglycemic reactions.

Mary Lu Rang, RN, MSN, CRNP

Kits, carts, and emergency care #2

In our intensive care unit, we've simplified storing and transporting emergency supplies. We use two small, mobile carts that roll right up to the patient's bedside. One cart holds supplies for starting any kind of line—I.V., arterial, total parenteral nutrition, Swan-Ganz, or cutdown.

This cart also holds arm boards, tape, alcohol wipes, dressing change kits, and povidone-iodine ointment.

The other cart holds supplies for gastrointestinal bleeding—nasogastric tubes, gastrointestinal tubes, saline bottles, large irrigation syringes, disposable underpads, and so on.

The carts save us time collecting supplies and carrying them to the patient's bedside. What's more, new staff and pool nurses can quickly find supplies in an emergency.

Linda P. Massimiano, RN

Ready for an emergency

When an emergency patient is admitted to our intensive care unit, we don't always have time to collect isolation equipment. So we now keep emergency packs in convenient places throughout the unit. The packs include isolation gowns, gloves, masks, goggles, and shoe covers.

Candy Sandal, RN, CCRN

Finding ECG leads quickly

In our crash cart, we keep the five electrocardiogram (ECG) lead clips attached to a stick figure that we've made from tongue depressors. The figure has a gel pad on each limb and one in the center for the chest. Keeping the lead clips on the appropriate gel pads allows us to apply them quickly and prevents cables from getting tangled.

Douglas Rutkowski, RN

ECG wires: No more tangles

In our anesthesia unit, we stick about 30 electrocardiogram (ECG) electrodes on the side of the workroom refrigerator. We snap replacement ECG wires onto these pads—this way, the wires don't tangle, and they're easily accessible too.

David C. Tonry, CRNA

Time-saver for thrombolytic therapy

We keep a "clot box" in the emergency department for patients who require thrombolytic therapy. This box contains everything we'll need during an infusion of a thrombolytic, from chewable aspirin to a heparin drip. Having all the medications and I.V. supplies in a central location decreases the time between identifying a patient with an acute myocardial infarction and treating him.

Sherri Reynolds, RN, CCRN, BSN

Gloves on the run

As a critical care nurse, I'm part of the hospital's code team. To save time, I carry a pair of nonsterile gloves in my pocket and put them on as I'm running to the code scene. I can immediately begin suctioning the patient, drawing arterial blood gases, or inserting a peripheral I.V. line.

Isabelle M. Brunelle, RN

Catchall for ECG paper

During a code, electrocardiograph (ECG) paper may end up all over the wet, soiled floor. But here's an easy way to keep the printouts neat: Tape a large bag to the side of the ECG machine to catch them. When the code is over, remove the full bag and replace it with an empty one. This way, it's also easier to find and cut strips needed for the patient's code sheet.

Margaret Farny, RN

Finding lines

When patients have multiple I.V. and pressure-monitoring lines, you may have trouble figuring out which line is which.

So color-code the lines. For instance, arterial lines can sport a piece of red tape, pulmonary artery catheter lines may have green tape, central venous pressure lines will bear yellow tape, and each medication line will have a different colored tape marker.

The coding system helps you find the line you need quickly, which is especially important in an emergency.

Carol Steinruch, RN

Heard but not seen

When several I.V. infusion pumps are running on our unit at the same time and one starts beeping, we're never sure which room the signal is coming from.

To save time and steps, we put a small piece of colored tape next to the call button of each patient who has a pump. We also put a piece of tape on the door of each room that has a pump.

When we hear beeping, we call patients in the marked rooms on the intercom to find out which controller is signaling us. Then we go right to that room.

Marsha Miller, RN

Solutions on ice #1

In our 10-bed cardiac/intensive care unit, we never know when we'll need to measure a patient's cardiac output with the thermodilution technique. To make sure we're prepared, we keep a 500-ml bottle of D_5W in our refrigerator. When we have to fill syringes for a cardiac output measurement, the injectate is already chilled and doesn't have to be iced.

The nurse who takes the bottle of D_5W from the refrigerator is responsible for replacing it. And we all check the bottles' expiration dates periodically.

Lorna E. Stern, RN

Solutions on ice #2

We had several patients on our unit recently with GI bleeding. We spent so much time doing iced lavages that we decided we had to be better prepared for them. So we put a few large bottles of normal saline solution in the refrigerator.

Now whenever iced lavages are needed, the solution is already cool. We just have to get the ice and replace the used saline solution with a new bottle.

Bonnie Handerhan, RN, BSN

Portable caddies

Instead of a centrally located I.V. tray or cart, we keep plastic caddies stocked with essential supplies in specific areas of our obstetrics/gynecology unit. We have a supply caddy in each birthing room, one in our main delivery room, one at the nurses' station medications area, and one stocked with special supplies on our nursery crash cart.

The caddies are two-sided with a central handle and are portable enough to be carried quickly to any area where they're needed.

Kate White, RN

Measuring made easy

If your patient has a pulmonary artery catheter and needs to have his cardiac output measured frequently, do you disconnect the catheter's proximal lumen hub from the I.V. tubing each time to inject iced saline solution? That's a time-consuming procedure. Instead, connect the hub to the I.V. tubing with a 3-way stopcock. Then, you can push the iced saline solution through the stopcock. You'll not only save the time of disconnecting the tubing, but you'll also decrease the possibility of contaminating the line or introducing air into it.

René R. Guild, RN

Airway innovations

In our emergency department, we've finally come up with a method for neatly storing oral airways. We hang them on a rack, which is simply a board with nails in it. Each airway hangs by its flanged end on two nails, appropriately spaced to accommodate the airway size. We mounted the rack near our monitors, where it's out of the way yet easily accessible.

Callie Sandquist, RN

Logging expiration dates

To make checking the expiration dates of your unit's stock medications simpler, keep a log. As soon as you receive new medication, record each drug under the month in which it expires. Then you can check the log periodically, and quickly and easily identify the drugs that have expired.

Geetha Eapen

Date with dots

Use colored dots to flag expiration dates, so you'll remember to replace out-of-date supplies. You'd use a different color for each month; for example, you might put a red dot on all supplies that will

expire at the end of June. If you want, you can also write the year on the dot.

L. Coughlin, RN, BSN

Minimizing cart chaos

Before passing medications, I make sure my cart is complete and organized. I check that I have different sizes of syringes and needles, medication cups, alcohol wipes, I.V. starter kits, tubing for I.V. piggyback medications, I.V. connectors, specimen cups, juice (for patients who prefer it to water), and a plastic waste bag. Being organized saves me trips to the nurses' station.

Irene J. Leonardo, RN

Keys to saving time

Because I administer medications on several units, I've color-coded the keys to the different medication cabinets. I place a colored stick-on dot on each cabinet and its corresponding key. This takes the guesswork out of matching the key to the lock.

Mary Regan Brakey, RN, MSN

Tight turnaround

In our busy emergency department (ED), we use a kitchen timer to help improve turnaround time and prevent discharge delays. Here's how: Because our hospital's policy requires that patients wait 20 minutes after receiving an antibiotic injection, we set the timer as soon as a patient has received an injection. Then 20 minutes later, the timer alerts the staff to discharge the patient. This prevents him from spending unnecessary time in the ED and serves as a helpful reminder to the staff.

Mavis A. Lowrey, RN, BSN

Free ticket to ride

When a patient is ready to be discharged from our ambulatory surgery center, we sometimes have trouble locating the person who's driving him home. The driver may have left the center "for a few minutes" and not yet returned.

So we developed a "freedom ticket" for the driver. The ticket thanks him for bringing the patient, tells him when to return to the center, and reminds him to check in with the receptionist. It also informs him that he may have to stop and have prescriptions filled for the patient. The driver signs the form and keeps the original—we have a copy for reference.

We now have fewer delays when we want to discharge our patients, and the drivers have some freedom during the waiting period.

Joan Macfadyen, RN, BS

Documentation: Skin stamp

Describing wounds and their treatment can be a time-consuming part of charting. I developed a skin documentation stamp to make the job easier. This stamp includes space for recording the location, size, and depth of the wound and for describing the tissue, drainage, and treatment. All the nurse has to do is fill in the blanks.

Roseanne M. Ottaggio, RN, CDE, MSN

Handy ruler

You can use your index finger as a tool for estimating wound size. Measure each section of your finger and remember its length. That way, you'll have a measuring aid that's always "handy."

Donna Edelmann, RN

Pocket timer

Ever wish you could set an alarm to remind you to check an I.V. line or look in on a patient? I carry a little parking meter timer with me for such purposes. The timer, which I pin to the inside of my pocket, can be set for any interval up to an hour.

Elke Trilling, RN

Pin point

I save time by fastening a safety pin to the handle of my bandage scissors. I don't have to look around when I need a sharp point, for instance, to puncture air holes in a new colostomy bag or to check extremity sensation during a neurologic exam.

Kathleen Porter, RN

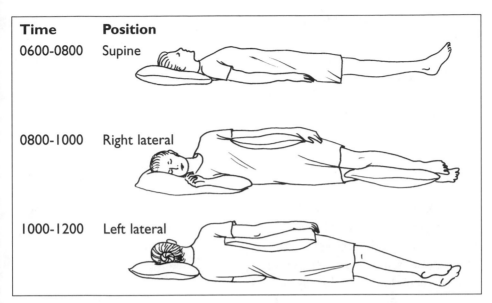

Time	Position
0600-0800	Supine
0800-1000	Right lateral
1000-1200	Left lateral

Right time, right position

In our busy unit, it's hard to remember the turning schedule for each patient confined to bed—and what his previous position was. To prevent confusion, I make a reference guide and attach it to the bed. The guide lists the time (0600–0800, 0800–1000, 1000–1200, and so forth) and position (supine, right lateral, left lateral) the patient should be in.

Mitzi A. Llamas, RN

One less needlestick

In the labor and delivery department where I work, we always draw an extra tube of blood for routine blood tests. We label the extra tube and put it in the refrigerator. If the patient needs a stat uric acid test during labor or a type and cross-match for an unplanned cesarean section, we can use the extra blood and not bother the patient with another needlestick. If we don't use the extra blood, we discard it after delivery.

Lana Carnithan, RN

Taking turns to prevent pressure ulcers

At the nursing home where I work, we prevent pressure ulcers in our residents by turning them every 2 hours. To be sure everyone on the night shift remembers to do this, I've developed a simple routine that has worked well.

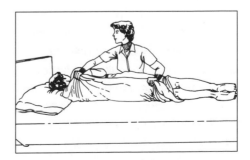

When the evening-shift nurses make their last rounds, they turn the residents toward the windows. At midnight, we turn them toward the doors; at 2 a.m., toward the windows; at 4 a.m. toward the doors; and at 6 a.m., we turn them on their backs.

Betty Bartz, RN

Tape to go

Try hanging a partially used roll of tape on your stethoscope. It's less bulky than a full roll, and it's a good way to keep some tape readily available.

Joan Grant, RN, BSN

Bandage supply unit

In the clinic where I work, we use adhesive bandages of many shapes and sizes. To save time, we store them in an 18-drawer box (the kind carpenters use for nails) and stick a sample bandage to the front of each drawer. Now, finding the right size and restocking all sizes are easy. We use the same kind of cabinet to store suture materials.

Jeanne Ralston, RN

Glucose testing strips

In the doctor's office where I work, we cut the costs of blood and urine glucose tests by cutting reagent strips in half. Even cut in half, the strip has enough reagent to give an accurate reading.

Donna Priestly, GN

12 ACTIVITIES OF DAILY LIVING

Closed curtains for privacy

Here's a way to ensure a patient's privacy during physical assessments, bed baths, or invasive procedures: Pull the curtains around his bed and join the ends with a hemostat. Now the patient can be assured that the curtains won't come open, reducing any anxiety he may have.

Dasha Pisarik Ziegler, RN,C, BS

Fresh as a baby

I keep a bottle of baby bath on our unit. It's a great substitute for shampoo or the perfumed soap that a patient may ask for but can't get at the hospital. Baby bath is inexpensive, smells good, and is a nice pick-me-up for a patient.

Colleen M. Hamilton, RN

Hair-washing help

Try this the next time you wash a bedridden patient's hair: Hang a new enema bag from an I.V. pole and place the patient's head in a wash basin. Then use water from the bag to wash and rinse.

Cindy Adams, LPN

Gentler grooming

Here's a faster, tangle-free way to apply no-rinse shampoo. First, place a double-thick 4" x 4" gauze pad over the head and through the bristles of a firm hairbrush. Then, pour the shampoo on the gauze pad and brush your patient's hair. Replace the used gauze pad with a fresh one and continue brushing to remove excess shampoo. This effective method gently picks up oil and debris. You can also wash sections of hair without wetting or disturbing an incision.

Terrilynn M. Quillen, RN

Hair-rinsing help

Washing a patient's hair can be a cumbersome process. A watering can with a long, slender spout—the kind used for houseplants—can help. Most hold enough water to rinse short hair, and the spout allows you to direct the stream of water. Also, the water coming from the spout has more force than that coming from sprayers or a cup, so the hair gets a good rinse.

Sue Nesmith, RN

No more tangles

An electroencephalogram may leave a patient's hair full of collodion or contact cement. I've found an effective way to get rid of this material without tangling his hair.

After removing the major buildup (using department procedure), apply a liberal amount of conditioner or baby oil to his scalp. Massage well, rinse, and run a comb through his hair. Then shampoo as usual.

This technique helps loosen the cement and allows you to wash your patient's hair painlessly.

Terrilynn Quillen, RN

Substitute suds

When we can't find shampoo to wash a patient's hair, we substitute the castile soap normally used for soapsuds enemas. Each packet contains enough for two washings. Castile soap lathers well and is gentler than bar soap.

Valerie Davis, LPN

Soaking up suds

If a shampoo board is uncomfortable, try putting an adult diaper under a patient's head to absorb the shampoo and water when you wash his hair. Position one leg opening of the diaper around the patient's neck to prevent the water from leaking.

Catherine Humphries, RN, BSN

Dry shampoo

Here's an easy way to help your patients keep their hair looking clean without washing it: Work a little talcum or baby powder through their hair, then comb or brush it out. The powder will absorb most of the oil, so their hair will look and feel cleaner.

Claire E. Mendenhall, RN

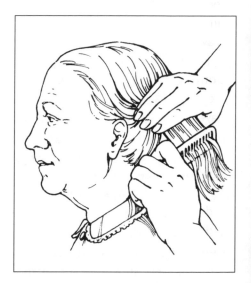

A hair bin

One of my biggest problems in caring for my bedridden mother after her stroke was how to wash her hair without getting water all over the bed and floor or causing her unnecessary discomfort. A plastic, stackable vegetable bin (with a half-circle cut out from the rim on one side), a large plastic trash bag, one heavy towel, and one hand towel helped solve the problem.

I put the plastic trash bag under

my mother's head and the heavy towel over the bag. Then I padded the cutout section of the vegetable bin with the hand towel. I placed the bin under her head with her neck resting on the cutout section. To wash her hair, I poured a pitcher of warm water over her hair into the bin and applied shampoo. I removed and emptied the bin as needed. After rinsing, I removed the bin and dried her hair with the heavy towel.

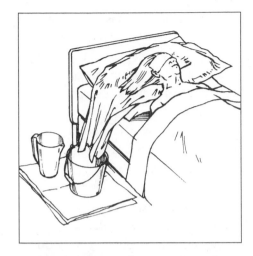

My technique works: While my mother got a refreshing hair wash, she stayed comfortable and her bed stayed dry.

Connie Davis, RN

Portable beauty parlor

If you've ever wanted to wash a bedridden patient's hair but couldn't find the plastic tray used for hair washing, here's a slick substitute. The materials to make it are always close at hand.

Open a bath blanket to its full length and roll it into a log. Fold the rolled-up blanket into a U-shape and place it inside a large plastic bag (such as those used for contaminated waste). Put the bottom of the "U" at the bottom of the bag. Then put the bag at the head of the bed with its open end hanging over the edge. The bag thus becomes a three-sided basin. Put a bucket on the floor under the open side of the basin to catch the water as it drains out.

Now position the patient with his head in the basin and his neck over the rolled blanket, and scrub away. The patient will enjoy the relaxing shampoo, and you'll love the job's ease. Best of all, the bed will stay dry.

Janice Petersen, RN

Ring around the collar

Make a washable cover for a patient's cervical collar by cutting a length of tubular stockinette (the kind used under casts) to fit around

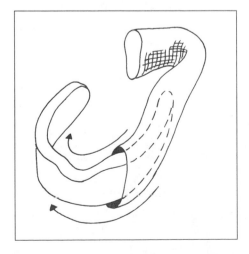

the collar. Nine inches of 3"-wide stockinette will fit a medium adult collar; 9"of 4"-wide stockinette will fit a large adult collar. Put one cover on the collar before the patient is discharged and give him an extra one to take home. The collar will stay cleaner with this cover.

Dorothy Fisk, RN

Coming clean

A patient who wears a shoulder immobilizer may develop body odor because he can't wash under his arm or apply deodorant. To solve the problem, give him this tip:

Drape a damp, soapy washcloth around a tongue blade. Carefully place the washcloth and tongue blade under the armpit. Remove the tongue blade, and clean the armpit by gently pulling the washcloth back and forth. Rinse and dry the same way.

Then apply spray or roll-on deodorant to a clean, dry washcloth. Fold the washcloth in half, drape it on a tongue blade, and place it under the armpit. Remove the tongue blade, but leave the washcloth under the armpit to absorb moisture and control odor.

Gladys M. Thorsell, RN

A kitchen remedy

To help keep bedridden patients dry, comfortable, and odor-free between baths, we dust them with baking soda. It doesn't cake in their skin folds the way bath powder sometimes does. Also, it has no fragrance, so patients who don't want a perfumed scent aren't offended—they just feel fresh and clean.

Alice Virant, RN

Body casts: Brushing away odors

Here's what I do to keep the perineal edge on a patient's body (or spica) cast odor-free. I place the patient on his abdomen or side and apply a thin layer of toothpaste to the perineal edge of the cast. I work the toothpaste into the cast with a toothbrush, leave it on for 20 minutes, wipe off the excess, then use a hair dryer on a low setting to dry the cast.

Sonja Jones, RN

A body (odor) guard

How can you help a patient who suffers from body odor that defies soap and deodorants? Try washing his offending feet or underarms with mouthwash, full strength or diluted. Or if the area's difficult to wash (a clenched fist, for example), just gently press a mouthwash-soaked washcloth against it for 10 to 30 minutes, then pat dry—no rinsing needed.

Suzanne D. Shutze, RN, CCRN

Clever cover for casts

A patient can shower or bathe without getting his cast wet if you cover the cast with clear plastic wrap. Secure the wrap with a piece of panty hose.

Ann Cunningham, RN

PICC protector

Long, plastic bags that hold disposable cups make great protectors for peripherally inserted central catheters (PICCs) when a patient takes a shower. Cut off both ends of the bag according to the size of your patient's arm, place his arm inside the plastic sleeve, and tape the plastic at both ends. This enables you to keep the PICC dry without applying tape to the patient's skin.

Julia Helen Sheville, RN

Keeping a heparin lock dry

If a patient has a heparin lock in his hand or wrist, place a latex glove on his hand to keep the heparin lock dry in the shower. Secure the glove at the patient's wrist with a piece of water-resistant tape.

Tina L. Kippes, RN

Sealed with a glove

Giving a tub bath to a patient who has an I.V. or heparin lock can be tricky, especially if the insertion site is above the wrist. To keep the site dry, I slide the patient's arm into a plastic bag. (Wastebasket liners work well.) I ask him to extend his hand to make sure he can move his fingers. Then I cut the fingers off a rubber examination glove and slide the glove over the plastic liner to cover the insertion site. This forms a seal without putting too much pressure on the arm.

Dorene Hunt, RN

Shower apparel

If a patient with a suprapubic or lower-abdominal dressing is allowed to take a shower, he'll need to keep the dressing dry. Here's what you can do:

Cut the end off a large plastic bag, then place the bag over the patient's head and pull it down so that it's covering the dressing. Gather together the excess top and bottom portions of the bag, and secure the bag by wrapping tape around his waist.

Now the patient can shower without worrying about his dressing.

Sujitra Vibulbhan, RN, BS

Convenient shower caddy

I had to spend a few days in the hospital as a patient—on crutches. Because I didn't have any free hands, I had a difficult time carrying my bath items to the shower. So here's what I did to solve the problem:

I removed the adhesive-backed bag from my bedside stand and filled it with my bath items. I could easily hold onto it while I used my crutches to get to the shower. Once there, I stuck the bag to the shower rail so the soap and shampoo were within my reach.

The bag worked great because I

could carry everything to the shower in one trip—and I didn't have to worry about dropping individual items.

Joyce Rambo, LPN

Staying afloat
When elderly patients can't tolerate showers, try bathing them on an inflatable air mattress in the bathtub. They'll be more comfortable, especially if they have pressure ulcers or bony prominences.

Jane Mooney, CNA-CMT

Sponging off
For patients who have one arm or one hand immobilized, using a washcloth is difficult. A sponge is easier for such patients to handle. It fits right into the hand, can be wrung out easily, and doesn't require folding as a washcloth does. Patients feel more independent when they give themselves sponge baths.

A sponge is also effective for arthritic patients, since the squeezing action helps loosen up stiff joints.

Vicki Prechenenko, RN

Quick cleanup for patients
I leave a small container of prepackaged towelettes on a patient's bedside table. That way, he can easily reach them to clean his hands before meals or after using the bedpan.

Karen Fleming, LPN

Tongue depressors in hand
Some of my long-term care patients have such severe hand contractures that cleaning their hands is painful for them and difficult for me. To make the job easier and less painful, I wrap some gauze around four separate tongue depressors. Using two of the depressors and some soap and water, I gently insert them into the patient's fist to clean the insides of his fingers and palm. I use another depressor to dry the area. With the last depressor, I apply medicated powder.

Cleaning the hands this way helps prevent odor and infection without too much discomfort for the patient.

Fe Perez, RN

Mouthwash as a freshener
Mouthwash works well as a final mouth rinse after a patient has used his emesis basin. The mouthwash also freshens the emesis basin by reducing any foul odor.

Mary Solomon, RN

Rinsing through a straw
One of my quadriplegic patients devised this method to avoid having toothpaste run down his chin while rinsing. After I brushed his teeth, he used a straw to draw up his rinse water—then he returned the water back through the straw into the emesis basin.

By not spitting into the emesis

basin, he avoided spills and had more control over rinsing.

Teresa M. Jewett, RN,C

Oral hygiene, just a squirt

If you need to provide mouth care for a patient who can't open his mouth very wide, try this: Fill an irrigating syringe with diluted mouthwash solution. Carefully flush his mouth with the solution as you suction with a tonsillar suction device.

Judith Reishtein, RN

Tongue tonic

Patients on ventilators often get a hard white caking on their tongues. To remove this caking, we gently scrub the tongue with a gauze pad moistened with a clear soda. Besides keeping the tongue pink and moist, the soda scrub leaves no unpleasant aftertaste.

Diane Atkins, RN

Close shave #1

If you have to shave a male patient but don't have shaving cream on hand, try using surgical lubricant

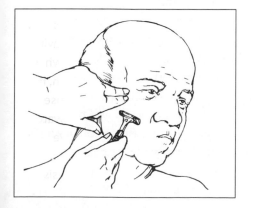

instead. The lubricant is clear, bacteriostatic, and water soluble. It allows you to give a careful and hygienic shave, and it's easy to clean up afterward.

Lawrence Beebe, SN

Close shave #2

If you need to shave a patient but don't have any commercial shaving cream, you *could* use plain soap and water. Often, though, this irritates the patient's skin. Instead, try this inexpensive, readily available substitute: Mix about a tablespoon of water-soluble lubricant with an equal amount of body lotion. This combination softens the beard, moisturizes the skin, and prevents irritation.

Sandra Meyer, RN

Brush a beard

In the trauma unit where I work, we see a number of patients with facial injuries. When those patients have beards, we have a problem. Sometimes we have to shave off the beard, but when it can be left on, we have a hard time cleaning the dried blood and debris from it.

What works best, we've found, is to gently scrub the beard with a toothbrush and a solution of warm water and hydrogen peroxide. The warm solution softens the crusted material, and the toothbrush allows us to scrub without applying too much pressure.

Ellie Franges, RN

Finger fresheners

I use toothpaste for my patients who get fecal material under their nails. I put some toothpaste on a soft child's toothbrush and brush their nails until they look and smell clean.

I also use toothpaste to clean cigarette stains from their fingers.

Ruby Tretreault, RN

Smooth skin cleanser

I use shaving cream to clean a patient's perineal area when he's been incontinent of stool. Shaving cream cleans thoroughly, is less abrasive than soap, and leaves the skin soft.

Mary J. O'Donnell, RN

Skin lotion potion

Cleaning dried fecal material from an incontinent patient is difficult. But a small amount of skin lotion applied with a soft cloth easily removes the material and prevents the dryness that soap can cause— even after rinsing with plain water. This technique is especially good for elderly patients and those with dry or fragile skin.

Elaine M. Neidert, SN

Peri-care(*fully*)

Some of the patients on our ortho-pedic unit are on complete bed rest for anywhere from several days to several weeks. I give the women perineal care this way:

I place a towel under the patient's hips and slide a bedpan under her, on top of the towel. Next I fill a clean container with warm soapy water, pour the water over the patient's perineum, and rinse with clear water. Then I remove the pan. (Applying a bit of lotion to the rim of the bed-pan beforehand makes it slide out easily, without pulling the patient's skin or causing the water in the pan to spill.) Finally, I dry the patient with the towel and remove the towel.

Nurses and patients both like this procedure because it's easy to give— and to receive.

Allyson J. Maes, RN

Soft and clean

For a quick, easy way to bathe a patient with dry skin, roll up one 6-ft-long towel (cut from a bolt of terry cloth—it's less expensive that way), one regular towel, and two washcloths. Wet the towels and cloths in warm water mixed with 2 oz of a lanolin-based soap, then put them into a plastic garbage bag to keep them warm until you're ready to use them.

Place the large towel over the patient's body and massage gently. Use the smaller towel for back care, one washcloth for face care, and the other for perineal care.

The bath is warm and relaxing. And because no rinsing or drying is needed, you won't irritate the patient's sensitive skin.

Diana Lehmkuhl, RN

Traction tip

To give patients the freedom to get themselves in and out of pelvic traction without your help, try this: Place an overbed table or two inverted trash cans under the weights at the foot of the patient's bed. When he lowers his bed, the weights fall gently onto the table and he can come out of traction. When he raises the bed, the weights lift off the table and traction is reapplied.

I devised this method when I was a patient in traction. It saved the nursing staff time and energy, and gave me some control over my care.

Regina S. Procopio, RN, CNOR

Relaxing rub

Here's a simple way to give your patients quick, relaxing back rubs: Hold a washcloth under warm water for a few minutes. (Make sure it doesn't get too hot.) Then squirt lotion on the cloth and gently rub your patient's back with it. The effect is very soothing.

Lucy Marie Wasowski, RN

Piercing tip

Remember to check patients with pierced ears for signs of infected earlobes. To prevent infection, clean the lobes with a solution of hydro-

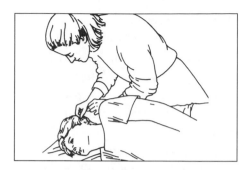

gen peroxide and water; loosen the patient's earrings if they seem too tight.

Patti Moore, RN

For the staff

A fantastic idea

To remove povidone-iodine or tincture of benzoin stains from your uniform, spray the stain with Fantastik spray cleaner. Then wash your uniform as usual—and the stain will disappear.

Janet Meyer, RN

Spotless suggestion

Iodine stains come out like this: Before machine washing, dip the affected area in milk, and rub gently. The stain will disappear.

Sister M. Monica, LPN

Fuzz busters

Do fuzzy little balls of lint decorate your old uniforms? If so, redecorate—with a safety razor. Just shave off the lint balls, and your uniform will look like new again.

Margery Lebel, RN

White again

Rust stains ruining your whites? Squeeze some lemon juice on the stains, sprinkle a generous amount of salt over the juice, and place the uniform in the sun until it's dry. Then wash as usual and—voilá!—your whites are white once again.

Etta M. Rosenthal, RN, BS, PHN

Stain 'n' scuff paste

To remove ball-point pen ink from your uniforms, wet the stained area and rub in some toothpaste. Rinse, then wash your uniform as usual.

Helen Bosch, RN

On-the-spot solution

Do you get ball-point pen ink spots on your uniforms? Here's a way to remove them. Wet the stained area, then pour a small amount of 70% isopropyl rubbing alcohol on the ink spots. Give the material a quick rub, and the spots will disappear.

Lucy Dalicandro, RN

Spot check

Here's another way to get rid of those seemingly indelible ink spots that adorn your uniform pockets—the products of uncapped pen points. Just saturate the spot with hairspray, then wash your uniform with your usual detergent. The result is a truly "spotless" uniform.

Cheryl Diorio, LPN

A pen pointer

If you like to keep two different colored pens on hand together but need a penholder that protects your uniform from unsightly ink spots, try this:

Measure and cut some used I.V. tubing about 20" from the drip chamber. Then cut the drip chamber in half. Cover the points of two pens with the drip chamber and wrap the rest of the tubing between and around the pens to prevent unraveling.

This penholder keeps your pens together and keeps the points covered. Best of all, no more ink-soiled uniforms to worry about.

Eva Tapoler, RN

Pocket protector

To keep pencils from smudging your uniform pockets, cover each pencil point with a rubber tip from a Vacutainer needle. The tips protect the pencil points and keep your pockets clean.

Norka Vélez Ramos, RN

Scuff stuff

When your white shoes get deep scuffs or scratches, coat the marks with white typewriter correction fluid. The fluid will fill in the scuff, permanently hiding and sealing it. And it's waterproof and durable besides.

Pamela R. Numbers, LPN

Shoes like new

Toothpaste will clean your white shoes. Just rub a dab over the scuff marks with a moist tissue or rag. Then polish with a dry tissue, and your shoes will look good as new.

Kathy Anderson, RN

Shoe biz #1

I keep my new duty shoes white by applying a coat of clear floor wax to them before wearing them. The wax helps prevent scuff marks, so I don't have to polish them as often.

Claire Mendenhall, RN

Shoe biz #2

To keep my old duty shoes looking like new, I use baby powder. First I apply white shoe polish as usual and wait until it's just about dry. Then I liberally sprinkle the powder on the shoes. When the polish is dry, I gently buff the shoes until they look as white and clean as new.

Mona Kuroki, RN, BSN

Shoe biz #3

Now that your shoes are white, what about the laces? To clean them, place them in a bowl or jar of warm water and add some dishwasher detergent. Agitate the laces in the solution, let them soak for 1 or 2 hours, then rinse and air-dry. Your laces will look as white and clean as your shoes.

Janet Widman, RN

Spotless suggestion

For spotless shoes, try wiping them with an alcohol prep pad. This removes dirt and smudges instantly.

Kathryn L.R. Bowling, Capt., USAF, NC

Soda for odor

To control odor in your duty shoes, sprinkle baking soda in them before putting them on each day. You can easily store the baking soda in a grated-cheese shaker or any container with large holes in the lid.

Susan Appleby, LPN

A tip with a ring to it

If you wear two rings on one finger, put the tighter of the two rings on last. Otherwise the looser ring could easily slip off when you're washing your hands or taking off disposable gloves.

Randi Greenberg, RN, BSN

13 POTPOURRI

Quick ID for dehydration

When protein is broken down in the body, one end product is urea, which is formed in the liver and eliminated through the kidneys. A key indicator of renal function, the blood urea nitrogen (BUN) level is normally between 10 and 20 mg/dl. Increased levels may reflect renal failure, severe muscle breakdown, hypovolemia, or excessive protein consumption.

The BUN level fluctuates widely when fluid balance is impaired. Dehydration, for example, causes it to increase because of hemoconcentration. Fluid overload causes it to decrease because of dilution. These fluid-dependent fluctuations make BUN ideal for identifying dehydration.

If you collect a blood sample for BUN testing, use a 5 to 10 ml red-top tube.

M.K. Gaedeke Norris, RN, CCRN, MSN

Serum potassium, handle with care

Normal potassium values range from 3.5 to 5 mEq/liter. Higher values may be associated with potassium-sparing diuretics, renal failure, Addison's disease, infections, trauma, burns, poorly controlled diabetes, and the use of angiotensin-converting enzyme inhibitors, such as captopril. Lower values may develop with congestive heart failure, renal disease, administration of excessive I.V. infusions without potassium supplements, malnutrition, and many potassium-wasting diuretics.

When drawing blood for a serum potassium level, use a 10- or 15-ml red-top tube. Draw the sample immediately after applying the tourniquet, and handle the specimen gently. (A delay or rough handling may cause hemolysis, which would falsely elevate potassium level.)

M.K. Gaedeke Norris, RN, CCRN, MSN

What can a sodium level tell you?

Normal serum sodium levels range

from 135 to 145 mEq/liter. Hyponatremia may occur from excessive diaphoresis, diarrhea, vomiting, burns, renal disease, hypervolemia, diuretic therapy, or GI suctioning. Diarrhea and vomiting can also cause hypernatremia if the patient loses more water than sodium; other possible causes of hypernatremia include aldosteronism and diabetes insipidus.

Symptoms of hyponatremia include apprehensiveness, lassitude, headache, cramps, and tremors. Hypernatremia is characterized by thirst, decreased urine output, dry mucous membranes, poor skin turgor, and changes in mental states, such as restlessness.

Draw a blood specimen using a 10- or 15-ml red-top tube. To avoid hemolysis, handle it gently.

M.K. Gaedeke Norris, RN, CCRN, MSN

A link between sodium and potassium

Normally, a patient's serum contains 90 to 110 mEq/liter of chloride. Hypochloremia is classically associated with sodium and potassium deficits. These low electrolyte levels could be related to several factors, including vomiting; nasogastric suctioning; chronic use of diuretics, bicarbonates, and steroids; respiratory acidosis; fluid retention associated with congestive heart failure; renal insufficiency; or metabolic acidosis.

In contrast, hyperchloremia can result from estrogen therapy, use of nonsteroidal anti-inflammatory drugs, anemia, dehydration, and renal disease. Signs and symptoms include rapid, deep breathing; muscle weakness; and stupor.

If you collect the blood sample, use a 5- or 10-ml red-top tube.

M.K. Gaedeke Norris, RN, CCRN, MSN

Counting white blood cells

A white blood cell (WBC) count with differential measures five types of WBCs (leukocytes)—neutrophils, lymphocytes, monocytes, eosinophils, and basophils—and tells if they're mature. The results are expressed as percentages based on a 100-cell sample, or as absolute numbers to indicate the number of WBCs per cubic millimeter of blood.

Neutrophils, the most plentiful type of WBC, kill and digest bacteria. (Immature neutrophils, called bands, also increase during overwhelming infection.) Lymphocytes, the second most plentiful type, produce antibodies. Monocytes work much like neutrophils, killing and digesting bacteria. Unlike neutrophils, however, monocytes quickly leave the circulation after the bone marrow releases them and enter tissue, where they're called macrophages.

Eosinophils, which play a major role in allergic conditions and parasitic infections, are phagocytes that consume antigen–antibody complexes. Basophils release histamines in an inflammatory response, such as an allergic reaction.

If you collect a blood sample for a WBC count with differential, use a 7-ml lavender-top tube.

M.K. Gaedeke Norris, RN, CCRN, MSN

Immature red blood cells

Reticulocytes are immature red blood cells (RBCs). Released from the bone marrow, they circulate for 24 to 48 hours while they mature. For men, normal reticulocyte counts range from 0.5% to 1.5% of the total RBC count. The range for women is 0.5% to 2.5%, with higher counts during pregnancy. An elevated count would indicate that the bone marrow is compensating for blood loss by releasing more young RBCs.

Decreased counts may occur from radiation therapy or chemotherapy—treatments that depress bone marrow function. Because of hemodilution, counts may be falsely low if the specimen is drawn from an arm that's receiving I.V. fluids.

If you're drawing the blood specimen, use a 7-ml lavender-top tube. Write the patient's medications on the laboratory slip because some drugs (such as chemotherapeutic agents, antipyretics, and azathioprine) can affect the results.

M.K. Gaedeke Norris, RN, CCRN, MSN

The weight of hemoglobin

The normal range for mean corpuscular hemoglobin (MCH), which is the weight of hemoglobin in a red blood cell (RBC), is from 26 to 32 picograms/red cell. Higher values accompany the same conditions that cause macrocytic anemias because larger RBCs contain more hemoglobin than smaller RBCs. For the same reason, low MCH values are consistent with microcytic anemias.

Mean corpuscular hemoglobin concentration (MCHC) measures the hemoglobin concentration in the average RBC. Normal values range from 30% to 36%. The MCHC value helps classify anemia by identifying RBCs as normochromic (normally colored, indicating normal hemoglobin concentration) or hypochromic (pale, indicating a low hemoglobin concentration).

The RBC indices are usually drawn as part of a complete blood count with differential. Use a 7-ml lavender-top tube and a needle that's no smaller than 20-gauge to prevent hemolysis.

M.K. Gaedeke Norris, RN, CCRN, MSN

Cold weather can alter platelet counts

Normal platelet values range from 150,000 to 300,000/cu mm. Lower values can be a sign of leukemia, vitamin B_{12} deficiency, folic acid deficiency, or severe blood loss. Other possibilities that may lead to a low platelet count are rheumatic fever, multiple myeloma, hepatitis, cirrhosis, and disseminated intravascular coagulation.

If you're drawing the blood for the platelet count yourself, use a 7-ml lavender-top tube. To identify possible interfering factors, review the patient's history for any drugs that might decrease the number of platelets or reduce their ability to function (e.g., antibiotics, thiazides, nonsteroidal anti-inflammatory drugs or other nonnarcotic analgesics, anticancer agents, and valproic acid).

Also keep in mind that cold weather, high altitudes, anabolic steroids, testosterone, and vigorous exercise can increase platelet counts.

M.K. Gaedeke Norris, RN, CCRN, MSN

Avoid false positives

Normally, serum contains less than 10 mcg/ml of fibrin split products (FSP) in a screening assay, or less than 3 mcg/ml in a quantitative assay. In disseminated intravascular coagulation, which causes massive clotting, FSP levels rise as the body breaks down the clots. If another clotting abnormality (such as thrombocytopenia) causes bleeding, however, FSP values may be normal. Other possible causes of elevated FSP levels include alcoholic cirrhosis, congenital heart disease, pul-

monary embolism, hemolytic transfusion reactions, and acute myocardial infarction.

Draw the specimen before giving heparin or you'll get a false-positive value. If you obtain the blood specimen yourself, use a blue-top tube provided by the laboratory. After drawing up the specimen, mix the blood with the tube's contents gently, to prevent hemolysis.

M.K. Gaedeke Norris, RN, CCRN, MSN

Clot-ability

Prothrombin time (PT), which determines the amount of time needed for a fibrin clot to form in citrated plasma, measures the clotting ability of Factors I (fibrinogen), II (prothrombin), V, VII, and X. It's the test of choice for evaluating oral anticoagulant therapy.

Normal PT ranges from 9.5 to 15 seconds. Certain disorders and drugs can prolong PT (e.g., liver or obstructive biliary disease, disseminated intravascular coagulation, vitamin K deficiency, indomethacin, phenytoin, quinidine, and aspirin). Antihistamines, corticosteroids, digitalis, and diuretics can shorten PT.

Using a 7-ml blue-top tube, draw the PT specimen in the morning prior to the administration of the warfarin dose, if indicated. Carefully fill the tube to the top; otherwise, the citrate in the tube will be disproportionately large for the amount of blood, artificially prolonging the clotting time. Gently invert the tube several times to mix the citrate with the blood specimen; place the tube on ice and send it to the lab immediately.

M.K. Gaedeke Norris, RN, CCRN, MSN

Evaluating APTT

Activated partial thromboplastin time (APTT) is a sensitive measure of most clotting factors in the intrinsic pathway, and is the test of choice for monitoring heparin therapy. Normal APTT values range from 25 to 40 seconds. Clotting disorders, liver disease, disseminated intravascular coagulation, leukemia, and vitamin K deficiency may prolong APTT. Extensive cancer may shorten APTT.

Using a 7-ml blue-top tube, draw a blood specimen in the morning, 30 minutes to 1 hour before the patient receives a heparin dose. Carefully fill the tube to the top; otherwise, the amount of citrate in the tube would be disproportionately large in relation to the blood specimen, artificially prolonging the clotting time. Gently invert the tube several times to mix the citrate with the blood. Place the specimen on ice and send it to the lab at once. Monitor the venipuncture site closely for bleeding or hematoma formation.

M.K. Gaedeke Norris, RN, CCRN, MSN

Albumin, a simple protein

Albumin, a simple protein, makes up more than half of total serum protein. It increases oncotic pressure (preventing capillary leakage) and carries hormones, fatty acids, and other insoluble substances in the bloodstream.

Besides protein deficiency, albumin levels help diagnose kidney, liver, and GI disease; cancer; and immune disorders. Normal levels range from 3.5 to 5 grams/dl.

Elevated albumin levels may accompany dehydration or multiple myeloma; decreased levels may indicate malnutrition, diarrhea, renal disease, an immune disorder, or metastatic cancer.

When drawing a blood specimen, use a 7-ml red-top collection tube. No food or fluid restrictions are necessary.

M.K. Gaedeke Norris, RN, CCRN, MSN

Broken-down old red blood cells

Bilirubin is a by-product of the breakdown of old red blood cells. Normally, it's processed or conjugated in the liver and excreted in bile. Direct (conjugated) bilirubin levels indicate how well bilirubin is being excreted after processing. Indirect (unconjugated) bilirubin levels help determine how well the liver is processing bilirubin.

Elevations in direct bilirubin indicate a biliary tree obstruction, which prevents normal elimination of conjugated bilirubin into the GI tract. Elevated indirect bilirubin levels indicate that the liver can't process bilirubin for elimination; the reason could be either liver disease or massive hemolysis that overwhelms the liver's ability to function. Depressed levels are less common and usually indicate iron deficiency anemia.

So, prior to obtaining a specimen, instruct the patient not to eat at least 4 hours before the test. (He may drink water, however.) If you draw the specimen for this test, use a 10- or 15-ml red-top tube. Handle the specimen gently—agitation can cause hemolysis, which would interfere with test results. Also protect the specimen from light, which causes bilirubin to break down.

M.K. Gaedeke Norris, RN, CCRN, MSN

Diagnosing through liver enzymes

Have you ever asked yourself just what AST and ALT are?

Both aspartate aminotransferase (AST) and alanine aminotransferase (ALT) are enzymes found in the liver and other body tissues. Normal serum AST levels range from 7 to 27 units/liter; normal ALT levels, from 1 to 30 units/liter. Higher levels indicate tissue damage.

Elevated levels are especially helpful in diagnosing cellular necrosis from liver disease. Other possible causes of elevated levels include hepatitis, cirrhosis, myocardial infarction, congestive heart failure, trauma, pulmonary embolism, pancreatitis, and extensive surgery. The higher the levels, the more extensive the damage.

Hold medications (especially hepatotoxic drugs) for 12 hours before drawing the blood specimen. Use a 7-ml red-top tube. To prevent hemolysis, handle the specimen gently. Note any interfering factors on the laboratory slip; aspirin, narcotics, and many antibiotics can alter test results. Draw serial AST and ALT levels at the same time each day (preferably in the morning) for consistent results.

M.K. Gaedeke Norris, RN, CCRN, MSN

Positive CRP is a negative

An abnormal protein, C-reactive protein (CRP) is produced by the liver in response to inflammation. It's not usually present in healthy people, so CRP results are normally negative.

Because CRP levels rise at the beginning of the inflammatory process, it's an even earlier indicator of inflammation than erythrocyte sedimentation rate. Test results help monitor the acute phases of rheumatoid arthritis and rheumatic fever. Other conditions that can cause positive CRP test results include lupus erythematosus, myocardial infarction, bacterial infection, and cancer.

Make sure the patient fasts for 4 to 8 hours (according to policy) before drawing the specimen; he can drink water, though. Use a 5- or 7-ml red-top tube.

M.K. Gaedeke Norris, RN, CCRN, MSN

Aid to food digestion

What does an amylase level tell you? Amylase, an enzyme produced primarily by the pancreas and saliva glands, helps with food digestion. Serum levels range from 55 to 190 international units/liter, or 25 to 130 units/liter.

Normally, amylase is excreted into the duodenum. In acute pancreatitis, however, it ends up in the peritoneal cavity, where it's absorbed by the lymph system and ultimately the bloodstream. Other conditions that raise amylase levels include bowel perforation, penetrating peptic ulcer disease, and mumps. Because advanced chronic pancreatitis causes extensive cell destruction, it lowers amylase levels.

Be sure to note on the laboratory slip any medications the patient is taking, including aspirin, azathioprine (Imuran), loop diuretics, narcotics, and oral contraceptives. Draw the sample in a red-top tube.

M.K. Gaedeke Norris, RN, CCRN, MSN

What's in a complement?

Serum complements are protein enzyme precursors that enable white blood cells and antibodies to move to inflamed or infected tissue to destroy foreign cells. Normally, the serum contains 41 to 90 hemolytic units. Complement assay levels usually decrease during autoimmune disease because constant inflammation consumes the enzymes. Conditions that increase levels include cancer, myocardial infarction, ulcerative colitis, acute rheumatic fever, and acute inflammatory reactions.

If you're drawing a serum complement level, draw the specimen in a 7- or 10-ml red-top tube. Be sure to send the specimen to the laboratory promptly, because test results may be affected by heat or the passage of time. Also, hemolysis (caused by handling the sample roughly) or recent heparin therapy can alter results.

M.K. Gaedeke Norris, RN, CCRN, MSN

Early detection for prostate disease

The normal prostate-specific antigen (PSA) level is less than 4 ng/ml in males age 40 or older and near zero for those who've had a prostatectomy. This test is frequently used to help diagnose problems of the prostate gland, including cancer, benign hypertrophy, and inflammatory conditions, so an elevated level doesn't specifically indicate cancer. For patients with a prostatectomy, the level is important in monitoring the progression of disease and the response to surgical, radiation, and hormonal therapies. Because PSA is found only in the cytoplasm of prostate cells, it's used as an early indicator of prostate cancer or its recurrence. Monitoring the rate of change in PSA levels is preferable to using a single measurement.

To collect a blood sample for PSA, obtain 5 ml of venous blood in a red-top tube.

M.K. Gaedeke Norris, RN, CCRN, MSN

How far will a red blood cell fall?

An erythrocyte sedimentation rate (ESR) simply measures the distance red blood cells (RBCs) in a whole-blood sample will fall in an hour. This is influenced by RBC volume, surface area, density, aggregation, and surface charge. Normal ESR ranges from 1 to 20 mm/hour for women, and 1 to 10 mm/hour for men. Elevated values mean RBCs are settling more quickly than normal.

An increase in plasma proteins such as globulin increases ESR by encouraging aggregation. Increased ESR values are common with inflammatory conditions such as rheumatoid arthritis, which raise globulin levels. Other conditions that can increase ESR include connective tissue disorders, cancer, ulcerative colitis, pneumonia, renal disease, and thyroid disease.

Hyperviscosity (high hematocrit) and low plasma protein levels slow ESR. Conditions causing low ESR values include mononucleosis and sickle cell anemia.

To draw the specimen, use a 7-ml lavender-top, a 4.5-ml blue-top, or a 4.5-ml black-top collection tube. Keep in mind, many drugs can affect the test results. For example, oral contraceptives, penicillin, and theophylline can increase ESR; aspirin, steroids, and quinine can decrease ESR.

M.K. Gaedeke Norris, RN, CCRN, MSN

ANA alert

In systemic lupus erythematosus (SLE) and certain other diseases, the body perceives its own cell nuclei as foreign and produces antibodies specific to the contents of the nuclei. Normally, antinuclear antibodies (ANAs) are present in serum dilutions up to 1:32. (This parameter may vary slightly, depending on the laboratory technique used at your hospital.) The presence of ANA in greater dilutions may indicate that the patient has SLE, some other autoimmune disease (such as rheumatoid arthritis or scleroderma), or an inflammatory disease (such as chronic hepatitis or mononucleosis).

If you collect a blood sample for the ANA test, use a 7- or 10-ml red-top tube.

M.K. Gaedeke Norris, RN, CCRN, MSN

Rest before TSH

Normal serum thyroid-stimulating hormone (TSH) levels range from 0 to 6 milliunits/liter by standard assay. To interpret abnormal levels, you must also know the thyroxine (T_4) level.

• Low TSH/low T_4 may indicate secondary hypothyroidism.

• Low TSH/high T_4 may indicate goiter or hyperthyroidism (thyroid hyperactivity suppresses TSH secretion).

• High TSH/high T_4 may indicate pituitary adenoma.

• High TSH/low T_4 may indicate primary hypothyroidism, thyroiditis, cirrhosis of the liver, or suppression of thyroid function by iodide-containing drugs or lithium.

Check with the doctor about holding medications, such as steroids, aspirin, and thyroid medications, before the blood specimen is drawn. The specimen should be drawn between 6 and 8 a.m., with the patient resting for 30 minutes beforehand; activity can change TSH levels. Use a 5-ml red-top tube, and note any medications the patient has received on the laboratory slip.

M.K. Gaedeke Norris, RN, CCRN, MSN

Serum T_4, what does it tell you?

Along with the other thyroid hormones, T_4 or thyroxine, is required for normal growth and development of the brain and bones and normal functioning of vital organs and other tissue. About 99.5% of T_4 is bound protein; the remaining 0.5% of the circulating T_4 is unbound, or free.

Normal T_4 values range from 5 to 12.5 mcg/ml. This laboratory test of the T_4 level measures both bound and free T_4. Use a 5- or 10-ml red-top tube to collect the blood sample.

M.K. Gaedeke Norris, RN, CCRN, MSN

Charting

Reporting an incident

When an incident occurs, do you ever wonder if you are documenting the incident adequately? Here are some tips to help you:

Only the person who witnessed the incident or first discovered it should file an incident report, and only that person should sign it. Anyone else with firsthand knowledge should file a separate report. Check your hospital's policy and procedure manuals for incidents that should be reported and the forms and procedures to use.

• Record the details in objective terms, describing exactly—and only—what you saw or heard. For example: "Found patient on floor beside bed" not "Patient fell from bed."

• Describe what you did at the scene, such as helping the patient back to bed, and your assessment findings. Also note any instructions you gave to the patient—for example, telling her to call a nurse for help if she wants to get out of bed again.

• Document the time of the incident, the name of the doctor you notified, and the time you notified him. Also notify your manager and have her review the form.

Incident reports should be retained by administration, not included in the patient's chart. Chart clinical details related to the incident (e.g., assessment findings and treatments). Just make sure the progress notes and incident report are consistent with each other.

Patricia Iyer, RN, CNA, MSN

Mistaken identity

To prevent ambiguity that could lead to treatment errors, remember these three cardinal rules about using abbreviations.

1. *Use only those abbreviations approved by your institution.*
Remember: Approved abbreviations differ from hospital to hospital, so you'll need to check the list in your unit or obtain one from your nurse-manager.

2. *Write legibly.* Even approved abbreviations can be misunderstood if they're not written clearly. And anything that's illegible to a staff member will surely stump a jury in a malpractice suit.

3. *Always explain abbreviations that can have more than one meaning.* Write out the potentially confusing term or word on first reference, followed by the approved abbreviation in parentheses.

Ellen Thomas Eggland, RN, MN

Charted course

On any busy unit, staff members may waste time looking for charts of patients who are off the unit for diagnostic tests. To cut down on frustration, we now place cards in the slot where the chart should be. These cards indicate where the patient has gone. Similar cards can be put on a turntable chart rack and held in place with magnets.

Juanita Gibbons, RN, BSN

Against advice

Your patient is angry and states he is going home from the hospital. What should you do? You can't force a mentally competent patient to stay in the hospital against his wishes. Find out why he wants to leave, and notify the patient's doctor. If the doctor isn't available, speak to the patient yourself. Make sure he realizes and understands the risks of leaving the hospital. Then ask him to sign the against-medical-advice (AMA) form, and document your conversation in your nurses' notes.

To guard against negligence charges, always document statements and actions reflecting the patient's behavior when he left. This will help if it happens that he was mentally incompetent or improperly supervised at the time.

If the patient refuses to sign the AMA form, document this refusal on the form—in his own words. Fill out an incident report if required by hospital policy.

Patricia Iyer, RN, CNA, MSN

Details, details

To avoid "broad-brushing" your narrative notes, always remember to include the following:

• Specific information including distances, quantities, time frames, and pertinent patient comments.

• Assessment findings that substantiate your interventions. Putting side rails down for a patient who's oriented x 3 and has good balance, a steady gait, stable vital signs, and no dizziness wouldn't seem inappropriate.

• Any specific precautions that other nurses should take.

Ellen Thomas Eggland, RN, MN

Tracheostomy care: Flow of facts

To save charting time when caring for a tracheostomy patient, we've developed an interdisciplinary tra-

cheostomy flow sheet. In eight one-line entries, we can document the type and amount of secretions and aspirate, frequency of suctioning and basic care, and presence of a cough. Each sheet has three identical sections, one to be filled out at the end of each nursing shift.

The flow sheet not only saves time, but also organizes information about the patient's care. Nurses and respiratory therapists can glance at the sheet for a quick assessment of the patient's condition and care during the previous 24 hours.

Mary Hartz, RN, BSN

Order by phone

If a patient requires immediate treatment and the doctor is not available to write an order, you may have no choice but to obtain a telephone order. Carefully follow your facility's policy for documenting a telephone order. Generally, you'd follow this procedure:

If time allows, have another nurse listen as the doctor gives the order. (Let him know someone else is on the phone.) At the very least, repeat the order, using the patient's name. For example, you'd say, "Doctor, you're ordering oxygen, 4 liters per minute, by nasal cannula and 40 mg Lasix I.V. bolus for William Perry, correct?"

Record the order on the doctor's order sheet as soon as possible. First, note the date and time, then write the order verbatim. On the next line, write "t.o." for telephone order. Then, write the doctor's name and sign your name. If another nurse listened to the order with you, have her sign the order too.

• Draw lines through any blank spaces in the order.

• Make sure the doctor countersigns the order within the time limits set by your facility's policy. Without his signature, you may be held liable for practicing medicine without a license.

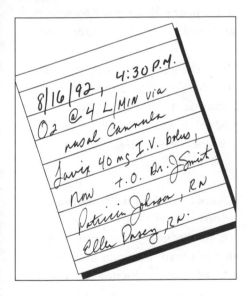

If you must document a verbal order, follow the same procedure, but substitute "v.o." (verbal order) for "t.o." Many hospitals no longer permit doctors to give verbal orders because of the high risk that a misunderstanding will lead to an error.

Patricia Iyer, RN, CNA, MSN

Write what you mean
When you document, you must make sure other caregivers know *exactly* what you mean—by giving precise times, amounts, sizes, and other characteristics. To describe dimension, you can use examples, such as "raised, pea-size cyst." Be concise but clear; reread your notes to make sure they're accurate. And always use correct medical terms and abbreviations approved by your facility; double-check if you're not sure.

Ellen Thomas Eggland, RN, MN

Protecting confidentiality
Who can see your patient's chart? Here are a few guidelines: In most cases you can't reveal confidential information—even to one of the patient's close relatives—without the patient's permission.

So don't release the chart to anyone who's not authorized, and don't give oral information about your patient to anyone, including visitors, police officers, or insurance investigators. If you're not sure how to handle a request for information, notify the doctor and refer the request to the appropriate hospital administrator.

However, the law requires disclosure of confidential information in certain situations—for example, those involving child abuse, public health hazards, and criminal cases.

Certain agencies, such as the Internal Revenue Service and public health departments, can also order disclosure of the information.

Who else might be authorized to see the chart? Here are a few guidelines:

• The patient may see his own chart, and health care workers directly involved in his care may see the chart.

• The next of kin or the patient's legally authorized representative may seek information if the patient isn't competent.

• The hospital may allow health care workers to review records for research, statistical evaluation, and education.

For details about rules and exceptions that apply in your state, check with your hospital's legal department.

Patricia Iyer, RN, CNA, MSN

Avoiding the defamation charge

How can you avoid being sued for defamation?

• Always make sure that what you say and write is an absolute fact, not an opinion.

• Discuss confidential information only with those who have an official reason to know. Remember: Fact doesn't justify a breach of confidentiality.

• Never allege another's negligence in an incident or editorialize about how an incident happened; just give the facts.

• Never write a derogatory comment about a colleague in the medical record, even if you believe it's the truth.

• When documenting your assessment of a patient, include only the objective findings; don't offer assumptions.

• Report an impaired colleague in good faith only—for example, after documenting examples of such behavior.

• If you give performance evaluations, justify all negative comments with examples that illustrate your point.

• Avoid using labels such as "hostile," "rude," "aggressive," "difficult," "combative," or "crazy" to describe people. Instead, describe their behavior; it will speak for itself.

Barbara E. Calfee, JD

Documenting a "harmless" medication error

If a medication error occurs, your documentation should be as objective as possible. Remember, you're recording the facts of your patient's care and treatment. You're *not* giving details about why the error occurred; leave that for the incident report. Your notes should include:

• Name and dosage of the medication and the time it was given

• Patient's response to the medication

• Name of the doctor and the time you notified him

- Any nursing interventions or medical treatment
- Patient's response to treatment
  Nancy B. Grane, RN, BS

Miscellaneous suggestions

Letting the air out
To obtain a good mask seal when using a bag-valve-mask device, I let air out of the mask until it looks about half full. This way, it molds to the patient's face better and less air leaks from around the mask during ventilation.

    John F. Brennan, Jr., RN, NREMT, CEN

Get a grip
Before putting a pediatric patient in a high chair, I place a rubber grip pad for opening jars on the seat. This prevents the child from sliding down under the tray. The grip pads also work well for geriatric patients.

    Teresa D. Leese, RN

Removing a stinger
To remove a bee stinger, use a credit card to flick the stinger off the skin or a pair of tweezers to pull the stinger out. Don't squeeze or pinch the skin because you may push more venom into the skin and cause more swelling.

    Myra Horn, RN

Odor busters
Bedpans and urinals can have lasting odors, so I fill them with water and add one or two of the effervescent tablets used for soaking dentures. These tablets can really make a difference.

    Deborah Gagnon Ellis, RN, MS

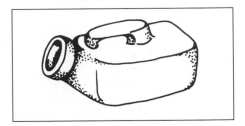

Staying pinned
To avoid losing my name pin when I wear it on my scrub uniform, I pin it right through the uniform to my bra strap. That way I can't take off the uniform without first removing the pin. I haven't lost a name pin yet.

    Pat Barta, RN

Pen pal
If your patient frequently loses pens, poke one in the top of his bedside box of facial tissues. Encourage him to return the pen to the box each time he's finished using it. This way, he'll always have a pen handy, and you won't have to keep bringing him new ones.

    Kathy Ptacin, RN

Compatibility of Drugs Combined in a Syringe

KEY

Y = compatible for at least 30 minutes
P = provisionally compatible; administer within 15 minutes
P(5) = provisionally compatible; administer within 5 minutes
N = not compatible
* = conflicting data

(A blank space indicates no available data.)

	atropine sulfate	benzquinamide HCl	butorphanol tartrate	chlorpromazine HCl	cimetidine HCl	codeine phosphate	dimenhydrinate	diphenhydramine HCl	droperidol	fentanyl citrate	glycopyrrolate	heparin Na	hydromorphone HCl	hydroxyzine HCl	meperidine HCl	metoclopramide HCl
atropine sulfate	▓	Y	Y	Y	Y		P	P	P	P	Y	P(5)	Y	Y	Y	P
benzquinamide HCl	Y	▓									Y			Y	Y	
butorphanol tartrate	Y		▓	Y	Y		N	Y	Y	Y				Y	P	
chlorpromazine HCl	Y	Y	Y	▓	N		N	P	P	P	Y	N	Y	P	P	P
cimetidine HCl	Y		Y	N	▓		Y	Y	Y	Y	Y	Y	Y	Y	Y	
codeine phosphate						▓					Y			Y		
dimenhydrinate	P	N	N				▓	P	P	P	N	P(5)		N	P	P
diphenhydramine HCl	P	Y	P	Y			P	▓	P	P	Y		Y	P	P	Y
droperidol	P	Y	P	Y			P	P	▓	P	Y	N		P	P	P
fentanyl citrate	P	Y	P	Y			P	P	P	▓		P(5)	Y	Y	P	P
glycopyrrolate	Y	Y		Y	Y	Y	N	Y	Y		▓		Y	Y	Y	
heparin Na	P(5)			N	Y		P(5)		N	P(5)		▓			N	P(5)
hydromorphone HCl	Y		Y	Y			Y		Y	Y	Y		▓	Y		
hydroxyzine HCl	Y	Y	Y	P	Y	Y	N	P	P	P	Y	Y	Y	▓	P	P
meperidine HCl	Y	Y	P	P	Y		P	P	P	P	Y	N		P	▓	P
metoclopramide HCl	P			P			P	Y	P	P		P(5)		P	P	▓
midazolam HCl	Y	Y	Y	Y	Y		N	Y	Y	Y	Y			Y	Y	Y
morphine sulfate	P	Y	Y	P	Y		P	P	P	P	Y	N*		Y	N	P
nalbuphine HCl	Y			Y			Y							Y		
pentazocine lactate	P	Y	Y	P	Y		P	P	P	P	N	N	Y	Y	P	P
pentobarbital Na	P	N	N	N	N		N	N	N	N	N		Y	N	N	
perphenazine	Y		Y	Y	Y		Y	Y	Y	Y					P	P
phenobarbital Na		N									P(5)					
prochlorperazine edisylate	P		Y	Y	Y		N	P	P	P	Y		N*	P	P	P
promazine HCl	P			P	Y		N	P	P	P	Y			P	P	P
promethazine HCl	P		Y	P	Y		N	P	P	P	Y	N	Y	P	Y	P
ranitidine HCl	Y			Y			Y	Y		Y	Y		Y	N	Y	Y
scopolamine HBr	P	Y	Y	P	Y		P	P	P	P	Y			Y	Y	P
secobarbital Na		N			N						N					
sodium bicarbonate											N					N
thiethylperazine maleate			Y											Y		
thiopental Na		N		N			N	N			N				N	

midazolam HCl	morphine sulfate	nalbuphine HCl	pentazocine lactate	pentobarbital Na	perphenazine	phenobarbital Na	prochlorperazine edisylate	promazine HCl	promethazine HCl	ranitidine HCl	scopolamine HBr	secobarbital Na	sodium bicarbonate	thiethylperazine maleate	thiopental Na	
Y	P	Y	P	P	Y		P	P	P	Y	P					atropine sulfate
Y	Y		Y	N		N					Y	N			N	benzquinamide HCl
Y	Y		Y	N	Y		Y		Y		Y			Y		butorphanol tartrate
Y	P		P	N	Y		Y	P	P	Y	P				N	chlorpromazine HCl
Y	Y	Y	Y	N	Y		Y	Y	Y		Y	N				cimetidine HCl
																codeine phosphate
N	P		P	N	Y		N	N	N	Y	P				N	dimenhydrinate
Y	P		P	N	Y		P	P	P	Y	P				N	diphenhydramine HCl
Y	P	Y	P	N	Y		P	P	P		P					droperidol
Y	P		P	N	Y		P	P	P	Y	P					fentanyl citrate
Y	Y		N	N			Y	Y	Y	Y	Y	N	N		N	glycopyrrolate
	N*		N			P(5)		N								heparin Na
Y			Y	Y			N*		Y	Y	Y			Y		hydromorphone HCl
Y	Y	Y	Y	N			P	P	P	N	Y					hydroxyzine HCl
Y	N		P	N	P		P	P	Y	Y	P				N	meperidine HCl
Y	P		P		P		P	P	P	Y	P		N			metoclopramide HCl
■	Y	Y		N	N		N	Y	Y	N	Y			Y		midazolam HCl
Y	■		P	N*	Y		P*	P	P*	Y	P				N	morphine sulfate
Y		■	N				Y		Y	Y	Y			Y		nalbuphine HCl
	P		■	N	Y		P	Y	Y	Y	P					pentazocine lactate
N	N*	N	N	■	N		N	N	N		Y		Y		Y	pentobarbital Na
N	Y		Y	N	■		Y			Y						perphenazine
						■				N						phenobarbital Na
N	P*	Y	P	N	Y		■	P	P	Y	P				N	prochlorperazine edisylate
Y	P			Y	N		P	■	P	P						promazine HCl
Y	P*	Y	Y	N			P	P	■	Y	P				N	promethazine HCl
N	Y	Y	Y		Y	N	Y	P	Y	■	Y			Y		ranitidine HCl
Y	P	Y	P	Y			P		P	Y	■				Y	scopolamine HBr
												■				secobarbital Na
			Y										■		N	sodium bicarbonate
Y		Y								Y				■		thiethylperazine maleate
	N			Y			N		N		Y		N		■	thiopental Na

Table of abbreviations

You may use these abbreviations, in health care facilities that approve them, to transcribe medication orders and document drug administration.

$\bar{a}$ before	cm centimeter	g, gm or GM gram	Ⓛ left
$\bar{aa}$ of each	comp compound	gr grain (quantity usually expressed in Roman numerals or Arabic fractions)	L liter
a.c. before meals	d day		LA long acting
A.D. right ear	/d per day	gtt drop	lb or # pound
ad lib as desired	D/C or dc discontinue	h or hr hour	m or M_x minim
A.M./a.m. morning	dil dilute	h.s. at bedtime	mcg microgram
aq aqueous (water)	disp dispense	Ⓗ hypodermic	mEq milliequivalent
A.S. left ear	DS double strength	I.M. intramuscular	mg milligram
A.U. each ear	D_5W 5% dextrose in water	in or " inch	mgtt microdrop or minidrop
b.i.d. twice a day	EC enteric coated	I.V. intravenous	ml milliliter
$\bar{c}$ with	elix elixir	IVPB intravenous piggyback	mm millimeter
caps capsules	et and	kg kilogram	MR x 1 may repeat once
cc cubic centimeter	ext extract	K.V.O. to keep vein open (patent)	NKA no known allergies
	fl or fld fluid		Noct. night

N.P.O. nothing by mouth	P.O. or p.o. by mouth	$\overline{s}$ without	t, tsp. teaspoon
NR no refills	pt pint	$\overline{ss}$ one-half	tab tablet
NS or N/S normal saline (0.9%)	q every	sat saturated	t.i.d. three times a day
NSS normal saline solution	q a.m. or Q.M. every morning	S.C. or SQ subcutaneous	tinct or tr tincture
¼ NS ¼ normal saline (0.225%)	q.d. every day	sec second	U unit
½ NS ½ normal saline (0.45%)	q.h. every hour	Sig write on label	vag, V., P.V. vaginal
O.D. right eye	q.i.d. four times a day	SL or sl sublingual	VO verbal order
os mouth	q3h, q4h, etc. every 3 hours, every 4 hours, etc.	sol solution	x times, multiply
O.S. left eye	q.o.d. every other day	sp. spirits	ʒ dram
OTC over the counter	QS quantity sufficient	SR sustained release	z or ʒ ounce
O.U. each eye	QNS quantity not sufficient	STAT immediately	> greater than
$\overline{p}$ after	qt quart	supp suppository	< less than
$\overline{p.c.}$ after meals	Ⓡ right	susp suspension	↑ increase
per by or through	R or PR by rectum	syr. syrup	↓ decrease
	Rx treatment, prescription	T, Tbs., tbsp. tablespoon	≈ approximately equal

Equivalent measures

The following table shows some *approximate* liquid equivalents among the household, apothecaries', and metric systems.

An agency or institution may acknowledge a particular set of equivalents as its official standard for exchange among systems. All health care professionals prescribing, dispensing, or administering drugs under such an agency's purview should abide by the established protocol. If no protocol exists, use the equivalent that is easiest to manipulate in any given computation problem.

HOUSEHOLD	APOTHECARIES'	METRIC
1 drop (gtt)	1 minim (M_x)	0.06 milliliter (ml)
15* or 16 gtt	15 M_x or 16 M_x	1 ml
1 teaspoon (tsp)	1 dram ($\mathfrak{Z}$)	4 or 5 ml
1 tablespoon (Tbs)	½$\mathfrak{Z}$	15 or 16 ml
2 Tbs	1 $\mathfrak{Z}$	30* or 32 ml
1 cup (c)	8 $\mathfrak{Z}$	240* or 250 ml
1 pint (pt)	16 $\mathfrak{Z}$	480* or 500 ml
1 quart (qt)	32 $\mathfrak{Z}$	960 or 1,000* ml
1 gallon (gal)	128 $\mathfrak{Z}$	3,840* or 4,000 ml

The following table shows some *approximate* solid equivalents among the avoirdupois, apothecaries', and metric systems.

AVOIRDUPOIS	APOTHECARIES'	METRIC
1 grain (gr)	1 grain (gr)	0.06* or 0.065 gram (g)
15.4 gr	15 gr	1 g
1 ounce	480 gr	28.35 g
1 pound (lb)	1.33 lb	454 g
2.2 lb	2.7 lb	1 kilogram (kg)

*Indicates the most commonly used equivalent when more than one is listed here.

Equivalent measures, continued

The following table shows some *approximate* solid equivalents between the apothe-caries' and metric systems.

APOTHECARIES'	METRIC
15 grains (gr) (¼ dram)	1 gram (g) (1,000 mg)
10 gr	0.6*g (600 mg) or 0.65 g (650 mg)
7½ gr	0.5 g (500 mg)
5 gr	0.3* g (300 mg) or 0.325 g (325 mg)
3 gr	0.2 g (200 mg)
1½ gr	0.1 g (100 mg)
1 gr	0.06* g (60 mg), 0.064 g (64 mg), or 0.065 g (65 mg)
¾ gr	0.05 g (50 mg)
½ gr	0.03* g (30 mg) or 0.032 g (32 mg)
¼ gr	0.015* g (15 mg) or 0.016 g (16 mg)
⅟₆₀ or ⅟₆₄ gr	0.001 g (1 mg)
⅟₁₀₀ gr	0.6 mg
⅟₁₂₀ gr	0.5 mg
⅟₁₅₀ gr	0.4 mg

*Indicates the most commonly used equivalent when more than one is listed here.

NANDA taxonomy I, revised

The North American Nursing Diagnosis Association (NANDA) endorsed its first nursing diagnosis taxonomic structure, NANDA Taxonomy I, in 1986. In 1989 and 1994, this taxonomy was revised. The revised taxonomy represents the currently accepted classification system for nursing diagnoses. The nine human response patterns and their definitions are: Exchanging: Mutual giving and receiving; Communicating: Sending messages; Relating: Establishing bonds; Valuing: Assigning worth; Choosing: Selection of alterations; Moving: Activity; Perceiving: Reception of information; Knowing: Meaning associated with information; and Feeling: Subjective awareness of information.

Pattern 1: Exchanging

1.1.2.1	Altered nutrition: More than body requirements
1.1.2.2	Altered nutrition: Less than body requirements
1.1.2.3	Altered nutrition: Potential for more than body requirements
1.2.1.1	Risk for infection
1.2.2.1	Risk for altered body temperature
1.2.2.2	Hypothermia
1.2.2.3	Hyperthermia
1.2.2.4	Ineffective thermoregulation
1.2.3.1	Dysreflexia
1.3.1.1	Constipation
1.3.1.1.1	Perceived constipation
1.3.1.1.2	Colonic constipation
1.3.1.2	Diarrhea
1.3.1.3	Bowel incontinence
1.3.2	Altered urinary elimination
1.3.2.1.1	Stress incontinence
1.3.2.1.2	Reflex incontinence
1.3.2.1.3	Urge incontinence
1.3.2.1.4	Functional incontinence
1.3.2.1.5	Total incontinence
1.3.2.2	Urinary retention
1.4.1.1	Altered (specify type) tissue perfusion (renal, cerebral, cardiopulmonary, gastrointestinal, peripheral)
1.4.1.2.1	Fluid volume excess
1.4.1.2.2.1	Fluid volume deficit
1.4.1.2.2.2	Risk for fluid volume deficit
1.4.2.1	Decreased cardiac output
1.5.1.1	Impaired gas exchange
1.5.1.2	Ineffective airway clearance
1.5.1.3	Ineffective breathing pattern
1.5.1.3.1	Inability to sustain spontaneous ventilation
1.5.1.3.2	Dysfunctional ventilatory weaning response
1.6.1	Risk for injury
1.6.1.1	Risk for suffocation
1.6.1.2	Risk for poisoning
1.6.1.3	Risk for trauma
1.6.1.4	Risk for aspiration
1.6.1.5	Risk for disuse syndrome
1.6.2	Altered protection
1.6.2.1	Impaired tissue integrity
1.6.2.1.1	Altered oral mucous membrane

1.6.2.1.2.1	Impaired skin integrity
1.6.2.1.2.2	Risk for impaired skin integrity
1.7.1	Decreased adaptive capacity: Intracranial
1.8	Energy field disturbance

Pattern 2: Communicating

2.1.1.1	Impaired verbal communication

Pattern 3: Relating

3.1.1	Impaired social interaction
3.1.2	Social isolation
3.1.3	Risk for loneliness
3.2.1	Altered role performance
3.2.1.1.1	Altered parenting
3.2.1.1.2	Risk for altered parenting
3.2.1.1.2.1	Risk for altered parent/infant/child attachment
3.2.1.2.1	Sexual dysfunction
3.2.2	Altered family processes
3.2.2.1	Caregiver role strain
3.2.2.2	Risk for caregiver role strain
3.2.2.3.1	Altered family process: Alcoholism
3.2.3.1	Parental role conflict
3.3	Altered sexuality patterns

Pattern 4: Valuing

4.1.1	Spiritual distress (distress of the human spirit)
4.2	Potential for enhanced spiritual well being

Pattern 5: Choosing

5.1.1.1	Ineffective individual coping
5.1.1.1.1	Impaired adjustment
5.1.1.1.2	Defensive coping
5.1.1.1.3	Ineffective denial
5.1.2.1.1	Ineffective family coping: Disabling
5.1.2.1.2	Ineffective family coping: Compromised
5.1.2.2	Family coping: Potential for growth
5.1.3.1	Potential for enhanced community coping
5.1.3.2	Ineffective community coping
5.2.1	Ineffective management of therapeutic regimen (individual)
5.2.1.1	Noncompliance (specify)
5.2.2	Ineffective management of therapeutic regimen: Families
5.2.3	Ineffective management of therapeutic regimen: Community
5.2.4	Ineffective management of therapeutic regimen: Individual
5.3.1.1	Decisional conflict (specify)
5.4	Health-seeking behaviors (specify)

Pattern 6: Moving

6.1.1.1	Impaired physical mobility
6.1.1.1.1	Risk for peripheral neurovascular dysfunction
6.1.1.1.2	Risk for perioperative positioning injury
6.1.1.2	Activity intolerance
6.1.1.2.1	Fatigue
6.1.1.3	Risk for activity intolerance
6.2.1	Sleep pattern disturbance
6.3.1.1	Diversional activity deficit
6.4.1.1	Impaired home maintenance management
6.4.2	Altered health maintenance
6.5.1	Feeding self-care deficit
6.5.1.1	Impaired swallowing
6.5.1.2	Ineffective breast-feeding

NANDA taxonomy I, revised

6.5.1.2.1	Interrupted breast-feeding
6.5.1.3	Effective breast-feeding
6.5.1.4	Ineffective infant feeding pattern
6.5.2	Bathing or hygiene self-care deficit
6.5.3	Dressing or grooming self-care deficit
6.5.4	Toileting self-care deficit
6.6	Altered growth and development
6.7	Relocation stress syndrome
6.8.1	Risk for disorganized infant behavior
6.8.2	Disorganized infant behavior
6.8.3	Potential for enhanced organized infant behavior

Pattern 7: Perceiving

7.1.1	Body image disturbance
7.1.2	Self-esteem disturbance
7.1.2.1	Chronic low self-esteem
7.1.2.2	Situational low self-esteem
7.1.3	Personal identity disturbance
7.2	Sensory-perceptual alterations (specify as visual, auditory, kinesthetic, gustatory, tactile, olfactory)
7.2.1.1	Unilateral neglect
7.3.1	Hopelessness
7.3.2	Powerlessness

Pattern 8: Knowing

8.1.1	Knowledge deficit (specify)
8.2.1	Impaired environmental interpretation syndrome
8.2.2	Acute confusion
8.2.3	Chronic confusion
8.3	Altered thought processes
8.3.1	Impaired memory

Pattern 9: Feeling

9.1.1	Pain
9.1.1.1	Chronic pain
9.2.1.1	Dysfunctional grieving
9.2.1.2	Anticipatory grieving
9.2.2	Risk for violence: Self-directed or directed at others
9.2.2.1	Risk for self-mutilation
9.2.3	Posttrauma response
9.2.3.1	Rape-trauma syndrome
9.2.3.1.1	Rape-trauma syndrome: Compound reaction
9.2.3.1.2	Rape-trauma syndrome: Silent reaction
9.3.1	Anxiety
9.3.2	Fear

Common laboratory tests

Hematologic tests

Erythrocyte sedimentation rate
0 to 20 mm/hour; rates gradually increase with age

Hematocrit
- Adult males: 42% to 52%
- Adult females: 38% to 46%

Hemoglobin
- Adult males: 14 to 18 g/dl
- Adult females: 12 to 16 g/dl

Iron and total iron-binding capacity (TIBC)

	Men	Women
Serum iron	70 to 150 µg/dl	80 to 150 g/dl
TIBC	300 to 400 µg/dl	300 to 450 µg/dl
Saturation	20% to 50%	20% to 50%

Red blood cell count
• Adult males: 4.5 to 6.2 million/µl of venous blood
• Adult females: 4.2 to 5.4 million/µl of venous blood

Reticulocyte count
0.5% to 2% of total RBC count

White blood cell count
4,100 to 10,900/µl

White blood cell differential
Adult values–
- Neutrophils: 47.6% to 76.8%
- Lymphocytes: 16.2% to 43%
- Monocytes: 0.6% to 9.6%
- Eosinophils: 0.3% to 7%
- Basophils: 0.3% to 2%

Coagulation tests

Activated partial thromboplastin time (APTT)
25 to 36 seconds

Bleeding time
- Template: 2 to 8 minutes
- Ivy: 1 to 7 minutes
- Duke: 1 to 3 minutes

Platelet count
130,000 to 370,000/mm^3

Prothrombin time
- Males: 9.6 to 11.8 seconds
- Females: 9.5 to 11.3 seconds

Whole blood clotting time
5 to 15 minutes

Common laboratory tests, continued

Arterial blood gases

PaO$_2$
75 to 100 mm Hg

PaCO$_2$
35 to 45 mm Hg

pH
7.35 to 7.42

O$_2$Sat
94% to 100%

HCO$_3$-
22 to 26 mEq/liter

O$_2$Ct
15% to 23%

Total carbon dioxide content
22 to 34 mEq/liter

Serum electrolytes

Calcium
4.5 to 5.5 mEq/liter (Atomic absorption: 8.9 to 10.1 mg/dl)

Chloride
100 to 108 mEq/liter

Magnesium
1.5 to 2.5 mEq/liter (atomic absorption: 1.7 to 2.1 mg/dl)

Phosphates
1.8 to 2.6 mEq/liter (atomic absorption: 2.5 to 4.5 mg/dl)

Potassium
3.8 to 5.5 mEq/liter

Sodium
135 to 145 mEq/liter

Serum enzymes

Acid phosphatase
- 0 to 1.1 Bodansky units/ml
- 1 to 4 King-Armstrong units/ml
- 0.13 to 0.63 BLB units/ml

Alanine aminotransferase (ALT)
- Adult males: 10 to 32 units/liter
- Adult females: 9 to 24 units/liter

Alkaline phosphatase
- 1.5 to 4 Bodansky units/dl
- 4 to 13.5 King-Armstrong units/dl
- Chemical inhibition method: Men, 90 to 239 units/dl; Women < age 45, 76 to 196 units/liter; women > age 45, 87 to 250 units/liter

Amylase
60 to 180 Somogyi units/dl

Angiotensin converting enzyme
18 to 67 U/liter (adults)

Aspartate aminotransferase (AST)
8 to 20 units/liter

Common laboratory tests, continued

Creatine phosphokinase
- Total: Men, 23 to 99 units/liter; women, 15 to 57 units/liter
- CPK-BB: none
- CPK-MB: 0 to 7 IU/liter
- CPK-MM: 5 to 70 IU/liter

Hydroxybutyric dehydrogenase (HBD)
- Serum HBD: 114 to 290 units/ml
- LDH/HBD ratio: 1.2 to 1.6:1

Lactic dehydrogenase (LDH)
- Total: 48 to 115 IU/liter
- LDH_1: 18.1% to 29% of total
- LDH_2: 29.4% to 37.5% of total
- LDH_3: 18.8% to 26% of total
- LDH_4: 9.2% to 16.5% of total
- LDH_5: 5.3% to 13.4% of total

Serum hormones

Aldosterone
1 to 21 ng/dl

Antidiuretic hormone
1 to 5 pg/ml

Chorionic gonadotropin
< 3 mIU/ml

Cortisol (plasma)
7 to 28 µg/dl in the morning to 2 to 18 µg/dl in the afternoon

Estrogens
- Premenopausal women: 24 to 68

pg/ml on days 1 to 10, 50 to 186 pg/ml on days 11 to 20, and 73 to 149 pg/ml on days 21 to 28
- Men: 12 to 34 pg/ml

Free thyroxine (FT_4)
0.8 to 3.3 ng/dl

Free triiodothyronine
0.2 to 0.6 ng/dl

Growth hormone
- Men: 1 to 5 ng/ml
- Women: 0 to 10 ng/ml

Insulin
0 to 25 µU/ml

Parathyroid hormone
210 to 310 pg/ml

Prolactin
0 to 23 ng/dl in nonlactating females

Thyroxine (T_4)
5 to 13.5 µg/dl

Triiodothyronine
90 to 239 ng/dl

Serum lipids and lipoproteins

Lipoprotein-cholesterol fractionation
- HDL: 29 to 77 mg/dl
- LDL: 62 to 185 mg/dl

Common laboratory tests, continued

Total cholesterol
- Ideal: < 200 mg/dl
- Borderline high: 200 to 239 mg/dl
- High: >240 mg/dl

Triglycerides
- Ages 0 to 29: 10 to 140 mg/dl
- Ages 30 to 39: 10 to 150 mg/dl
- Ages 40 to 49: 10 to 160 mg/dl
- Ages 50 to 59: 10 to 190 mg/dl

Serum proteins and pigments

Bilirubin, serum
Adult: direct, <0.5 mg/dl; indirect, ≤ 1.1 mg/dl

Blood urea nitrogen (BUN)
8 to 20 mg/dl

Creatinine
- Males: 0.8 to 1.2 mg/dl
- Females: 0.6 to 0.9 mg/dl

Proteins
- Total serum protein: 6.6 to 7.9 g/dl (100%)
- Albumin: 3.3 to 4.5 g/dl (53%)
- Alpha$_1$ globulin: 0.1 to 0.4 g/dl (14%)
- Alpha$_2$ globulin: 0.5 to 1 g/dl (14%)
- Beta globulin: 0.7 to 1.2 g/dl (12%)
- Gamma globulin: 0.5 to 1.6 g/dl (20%)

Uric acid
- Men: 4.3 to 8 mg/dl
- Women: 2.3 to 6 mg/dl

Serum carbohydrates

Fasting plasma glucose
70 to 100 mg/dl

Lactic acid
0.93 to 1.65 mEq/liter

Oral glucose tolerance test (OGTT)
Peak at 160 to 180 mg/dl, 30 to 60 minutes after challenge dose

Two-hour postprandial plasma glucose
< 145 mg/dl

Urinalysis

Routine urinalysis
- Appearance: clear
- Casts: none, except occasional hyaline casts
- Color: straw
- Crystals: present
- Epithelial cells: none
- Odor: slightly aromatic
- pH: 4.5 to 8.0
- Specific gravity: 1.025 to 1.030
- Sugars: none
- Red blood cells: 0 to 3 per high-power field
- White blood cells: 0 to 4 per high-power field
- Yeast cells: none

Common laboratory tests, continued

Urine concentration test
- Specific gravtiy: 1.025 to 1.032
- Osmolality: >800 mOsm/kg water

Urine dilution test
- Specific gravity: >1.003
- Osmolality: >100 mOsm/kg; 80% of water excreted in 4 hours

Urine chemistry tests

Amylase
10 to 80 amylase units/hour

17-ketosteroids (17-KS)
- Men: 6 to 21 mg/24 hours
- Women: 4 to 17 mg/24 hours

Creatinine clearance
- Men (age 20): 90 ml/minute/1.73 m^2
- Women (age 20): 84 ml/minute/1.73 m^2

Protein
< 150 mg/24 hours

Uric acid
250 to 750 mg/24 hours

Glucose oxidase
Negative

Ketones
Negative

Calcium
- Males: < 275 mg/24 hours

- Females: < 250 mg/24 hours

Phosphate
< 1,000 mg/24 hours

Sodium
30 to 280 mEq/24 hours

Chloride
110 to 250 mEq/24 hours

Cerebrospinal fluid

Glucose
50 to 80 mg/100 ml (two-thirds of blood glucose)

Pressure
50 to 180 mm H2O

Protein
15 to 45 mg/dl

Stool tests

Lipids
Less than 20% of excreted solids, with excretion of less than 7 g/24 hours

Occult blood
2.5 mg/24 hours

Urobilinogen
50 to 300 mg/24 hours

Index